D1531801

Child and Adolescent Mental Health Consultation in Hospitals, Schools, and Courts

Child and Adolescent Mental Health Consultation in Hospitals, Schools, and Courts

Gregory K. Fritz, M.D.
Richard E. Mattison, M.D.
Barry Nurcombe, M.D.
Anthony Spirito, Ph.D.

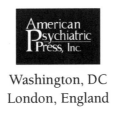

American Psychiatric Press, Inc.

Washington, DC
London, England

Note: The authors have worked to ensure that all information in this book concerning drug dosages, schedules, and routes of administration is accurate as of the time of publication and consistent with standards set by the U.S. Food and Drug Administration and the general medical community. As medical research and practice advance, however, therapeutic standards may change. For this reason and because human and mechanical errors sometimes occur, we recommend that readers follow the advice of a physician who is directly involved in their care or the care of a member of their family.

Books published by the American Psychiatric Press, Inc., represent the views and opinions of the individual authors and do not necessarily represent the policies and opinions of the Press or the American Psychiatric Association.

Copyright © 1993 American Psychiatric Press
ALL RIGHTS RESERVED
Manufactured in the United States of America on acid-free paper
96 95 94 93   4 3 2 1
First Edition

American Psychiatric Press, Inc.
1400 K Street, N.W., Washington, DC   20005

Library of Congress Cataloging-in-Publication Data
Child and adolescent mental health consultation in hospitals, schools,
    and courts / Gregory K. Fritz . . . [et al.].
        p.   cm.
    Includes bibliographical references and index.
    ISBN 0-88048-418-7
    1. Mental health consultation.   2. Behavioral assessment of
children.   3. Behavioral assessment of teenagers.   I. Fritz,
Gregory K., 1949–   .
    [DNLM: 1. Forensic Psychiatry.   2. Hospitals, Pediatric.
3. Mental Disorders—in adolescence.   4. Mental Disorders—in
infancy & childhood.   5. Referral and Consultation.   6. School
Health Services.   WM 30 C5351]
RJ503.45.C48   1993
618.92′689—dc20
DNLM/DLC
for Library of Congress   92-48975
                                                                          CIP

British Library Cataloguing in Publication Data
A CIP record is available from the British Library.

Contents

Affiliations

Gregory K. Fritz, M.D.
Professor of Psychiatry
Department of Psychiatry and Human Behavior
Brown University School of Medicine
Director of Child and Family Psychiatry
Rhode Island Hospital
Providence, Rhode Island

Richard E. Mattison, M.D.
Blanche F. Ittleson Associate Professor of Child Psychiatry
Director, Division of Child Psychiatry
Washington University School of Medicine
St. Louis, Missouri

Barry Nurcombe, M.D.
Professor of Psychiatry
Director, Division of Child and Adolescent Psychiatry
Department of Psychiatry
Vanderbilt University School of Medicine
Nashville, Tennessee

Anthony Spirito, Ph.D.
Associate Professor of Psychiatry
Department of Psychiatry and Human Behavior
Brown University School of Medicine
Director of Psychology
Rhode Island Hospital
Providence, Rhode Island

Introduction
What Is Consultation?

Psychiatrists and psychologists have functioned as consultants for decades to virtually every type of agency, institution, or professional group that deals with people. For children, the settings outside the mental health system where consultation is most often delivered are hospitals, schools, and courts. Consultation provides a psychiatrist or psychologist with an efficient means to help a larger number of children than could be reached via direct treatment only, and it serves to inject mental health expertise at critical points in the functioning of these other systems. In view of the magnitude of the need and the frequency with which psychiatrists and psychologists provide consultation, formal training in how to be an effective consultant has become an essential component of fellowship programs in both disciplines.

There is no single, universally accepted definition of the term "consultant." Webster's dictionary defines a consultant as "one who gives professional advice or services." In Europe, "consultation" is a term for seeking help; an individual "consults" a physician. Our definition is narrower: when working as a consultant, a psychiatrist or psychologist provides an expert opinion on a psychosocial problem to another professional in a discipline other than mental health. Under this definition, consultation differs from traditional, direct patient care in three important respects:

First, the patient does not request involvement of a mental health professional; the formal request comes from another professional. The child and the parents rarely instigate the request through the referring professional; more often, they acquiesce to the idea as put forth by the

| | **Content** | |
	Case	Program
Client or program	Case consultation	Administrative consultation
Consultee	Liaison; consultee-centered consultation	Systems consultation

Focus

Figure 1. Models of consultation. *Source*: Caplan 1970.

professional with whom they are working. Uncommonly, consultation will be undertaken even though the patient or parents are un-enthusiastic or resent it. This situation is in sharp contrast to the typical outpatient request for evaluation and treatment initiated by the parent, which has important implications for the nature of subsequent interactions, confidentiality, targeting recommendations, and so forth.

Second, a consultation request implies a question, a desire on the part of one professional for information from another professional who has expertise in a special area. However, in contrast to traditional medical consultation, where the issue is usually straightforward and clearly stated, the question behind a mental health consultation is often complicated. There are likely to be hidden or implicit questions that involve the consultee's own reactions, the relationship with the patient, and behavior at multiple levels. The psychiatrist or psychologist must clarify the various possible questions involved in the consultation request, and then respond to both the overt and implied questions.

Third, the consultant does not assume responsibility for the management of the person who is the focus of the consultation. A request for a consultation is different from a referral for treatment in that the consultee retains professional responsibility for the case. The consultee is free to accept all, part, or none of the consultant's advice. The consultant who responds to a consultation merely as if it were a treatment referral will find few subsequent requests forthcoming.

Although most consultant psychiatrists and psychologists would agree with the above definition and characterization of consultation, the potential remains for considerable variation in consultation approaches. Medical consultation represents a traditional model, exemplified when a general practitioner consults a cardiologist about management of a patient's complicated arrhythmia. The cardiologist reviews the medical record, the cardiograms, and other laboratory data, examines the patient, and suggests a course of action. Frequently, the entire process is incorporated in written notes between the two physicians, without further dialogue. The cardiologist focuses only on the particular patient and the specific questions, answering them factually and as directly as possible. Whether the general practitioner has adequate knowledge of cardiology, a good relationship with the patient, interest and resources sufficient to carry out the recommendations, and so forth are issues not generally addressed in the cardiologist's consultation.

The influence of the community mental health movement in the 1960s and 1970s changed the way mental health professionals view consultation. An important tenet of the movement was that psychiatrists, psychologists, and social workers based in the community mental health center should help professionals in various caretaking agencies (e.g., police, medical staff, educators, welfare workers, clergy, and probation officers) to work more effectively with their clients. Consultation services to increase the psychological sophistication of the professionals working in the various community agencies were legislatively mandated as essential components of federally funded community mental health systems. With consultation, it was argued, agencies could form a better support network, prevent more serious psychological dysfunction, and promote optimal use of mental health resources. A decade of experience with mental health consultation was most clearly conceptualized in the writings of Caplan (1962, 1970). Although others (Berlin 1964; Tarnow and Gutstein 1982) have described models of consultation, Caplan's descriptions of various types of consultation embrace most of the possibilities.

Caplan proposes that two factors distinguish four basic types of consultation: *focus* and *content*. The focus, meaning the goal to which a consultant attends, can be either a specific case or program that is problematic, or it can be the consultee himself or herself. The content refers to the material that is discussed during the consultation. It can be individual cases with which the consultee is working or a program, service, or unit for which the consultee has administrative responsibility. The four possible combinations are illustrated in Figure 1.

Case consultation most closely approaches traditional medical consultation. Its purpose is to help the consultee find the most effective way to manage a particular case with which he or she is having difficulty. This form of consultation entails direct examination of the child by the consultant, specific and active recommendations, and only a secondary interest in carryover to the consultee's other cases. *Administrative consultation* is similar to case consultation except that an aspect of a program (e.g., recruitment, organization, or utilization) rather than an individual case is the content being discussed. Both of these forms of consultation are time-limited: once the issue prompting the request is addressed, the consultation is completed, although the door may be left open for future consultations.

In *consultee-centered consultation,* the focus is on improving the ability of the consultees to deal with the psychosocial problems encountered in their ongoing work. The particular case under discussion is viewed as "grist for the mill" that allows the consultant to understand the interpersonal difficulties and intrapsychic conflicts that impede the consultee's effectiveness. Whether the content is particular cases or problems in developing and running a program, the consultant seeks to develop a continuing relationship with the consultee. This form of consultation has many features in common with psychotherapy: It involves an interpersonal assessment of the consultee's anxiety and defenses; it relies on the strength of the consultant-consultee relationship; and confidentiality is essential. Consultee-centered consultation differs from psychotherapy in that the consultant-consultee relationship is one between equals and the method of change is indirect, relying on the metaphor of the case rather than a direct discussion of the consultee's personal history, dynamics, and so forth. Consultee-centered consultation requires a commitment to regular meetings. It entails various stages, including a period of preparation, the negotiation of a contract, a period of problem-solving work, and a termination phase. Like successful psychotherapy, effective consultee-centered consultation leaves the consultee better able to meet future challenges.

Examples of consultee-centered consultation in the medical setting would include a liaison relationship with a subspecialty clinic or a regular ward meeting with pediatric nurses. In the school system, a weekly meeting with health teachers to discuss issues involved in an AIDS/sex education program or a regular consultation with guidance counselors would constitute consultee-centered consultation. A parallel in the legal system would be consultation to a discussion group of family court judges to increase their psychological understanding or consulting with Legal Aid attorneys about adolescent issues.

In practice, the application of the consultee-centered model in its pure form is problematic. First, professionals in a hospital or a school are unlikely to view their own intrapsychic conflicts as the source of most of the psychosocial problems they encounter working with particular children. Thus, true "informed consent" for consultee-centered consultation is difficult to arrange in a satisfactory contract. When the consultees want tangible help with challenging children but the consultant is interested in consultees' professional growth, frustration and misunderstanding on both sides are the likely results.

Second, consultation not focused on particular children is hard to fund. Financial support can take various forms (e.g., clinical revenue, fee-for-service, and institutional stipends), but only a wealthy and sophisticated institution is likely to see the value of ongoing consultation that is focused on professional development.

Third, despite the emphasis on an egalitarian relationship, consultee-centered consultation runs the risk of turning into a colonial endeavor in which a mental health "missionary" brings true religion to "heathens" in other disciplines. It can be difficult to contain the discussion of personal psychodynamics within the metaphor of a particular case and to prevent the consultation from becoming psychotherapy. Transference feelings regarding the knowledgeable, powerful (or weird and hostile) consultant do develop but are difficult to deal with within the confines of the consultant relationship.

Last, consultee-centered consultation in any of its forms is hard to evaluate. There is no "product," little accountability, and, at best, only gradual and subtle changes in the consultees. Even an effective liaison program in a hospital, for example, is difficult to describe to skeptical administrators beyond testimonials of the participants. In the 1970s, the community mental health movement oversold the potential of consultation and did little in the way of outcome evaluation. Partially as a result of this overselling, there is today considerably less interest in the "pure form" of consultee-centered consultation within the medical, educational, or legal systems.

The authors' independent experience in three different settings leads to the conclusion that case consultation is the most viable means of contributing mental health expertise to a non–mental health system. Other models currently can be applied less frequently (liaison in the medical or school setting) or seldom (consultee-centered consultation with judges or lawyers). A model of consultation that does not include direct evaluation of the child and specific recommendations from the consultant is poorly received in most institutions these days.

Recognizing the primacy of case consultation does not mean that there is no current role for mental health professionals in enhancing the skills of medical pediatric staff, educators, and legal professionals. Psychiatrists and psychologists can be helpful in educating the professionals with whom they consult, increasing their sensitivity to psychosocial issues, facilitating resolution of conflicts within the system, and contributing to organizational solutions that improve the care children receive in the system. Opportunity for ongoing, indirect consultation usually arises out of a series of successful case consultations. The consultant's involvement in the expanded, indirect activities should not be expected to remove the need for further case consultation, nor should case consultation be viewed as only a means to the "real" end, that of changing the consultees or the system itself. Mental health professionals with consultative skills, interest in the functioning of professionals in other disciplines, and a willingness to work in different settings will always be needed to help in the comprehensive care of children. The chapters that follow are intended to help the psychiatrist or psychologist be an effective case consultant in a hospital, a school, or a court of law, as well as a practical-minded educator sought by non-mental health professionals to help them improve their skills in working with children and adolescents.

Gregory K. Fritz, M.D.

REFERENCES

Berlin IN: Learning mental health consultation: history and problems. Mental Hygiene 48:257–266, 1964

Caplan G: Types of mental health consultation. Am J Orthopsychiatry 33:470–481, 1963

Caplan G: The Theory and Practice of Mental Health Consultation. New York, Basic Books, 1970

Tarnow JD, Gutstein SE: Systemic consultation in a general hospital. Int J Psychiatry Med 12:161–185, 1982

PEDIATRIC CONSULTATION

Gregory K. Fritz, M.D.
Anthony Spirito, Ph.D.

Section I: Pediatric Consultation

Chapter One
The Hospital: An Approach to Consultation
  A. Definitions: consultation, liaison, and psychosomatic medicine
  B. Historical background
  C. The hospital system
      1. Types of hospitals
      2. System characteristics
      3. Previous consultation
  D. Professional staff on a pediatric ward
      1. Pediatricians
      2. House staff
      3. Nurses
      4. Social workers
      5. Child life workers
      6. Other staff members
  E. References

Chapter Two
The Process of Consultation on a Pediatric Unit
  A. Intake
  B. Preinterview steps
      1. Determining the reason for referral
      2. Preparation of the patient and family
      3. Further preliminary steps
  C. Parent interview
  D. Evaluation of the child
      1. Building an alliance
      2. The interview
      3. Mental status and physical examination
  E. Other information
  F. Confidentiality
  G. Initial recommendations
  H. Consultation report
  I. Summary
  J. References

CHAPTER ONE

The Hospital: An Approach to Consultation

Gregory K. Fritz, M.D.

A s many as 4 million children and adolescents will be hospitalized this year. A significant percentage will have coexisting psychiatric disorders, regressive symptoms in reaction to hospitalization, stress responses that exacerbate the illness, behavior patterns that complicate or impede treatment, or medication side effects or interactions. Many of their families will have difficulty adjusting to or coping with the children's physical disorder. Though the proportion of pediatric patients needing mental health evaluation and intervention is debated, it is clearly large and routinely underestimated. A major function of mental health professionals in pediatrics is providing consultation and liaison services. This chapter provides an overview of the process, beginning with the special nature and qualities of hospital systems and pediatric practice and the characteristics of pediatricians and other professionals who care for children in the hospital.

A. DEFINITIONS: CONSULTATION, LIAISON, AND PSYCHOSOMATIC MEDICINE

Caplan (1970) described four models of mental health consultation in his influential writings. In the medical setting, psychiatrists and psychologists are primarily involved in what Caplan termed "patient-centered" consultation. At the request of the attending physician, the consultant provides an opinion regarding the care of a particular patient—usually after evaluating the patient directly. Consultation is distinguished from *liaison* work, in which the focus is on the nonpsychiatric professionals rather than the patient. Such work is termed "consultee-centered" consultation in Caplan's schema. In a liaison capacity, the mental health professional develops an ongoing, collaborative relationship with a group of health care professionals and seeks to enhance their psychosocial understanding, sensitivity, and clinical skills. Liaison thus serves both an educational and a supportive function for consultees. In contrast to consultation, individual patients benefit only indirectly and secondarily from liaison work. Over the years, consultation and liaison have each been advocated as the single appropriate way for psychiatrists and psychologists to interact with the medical system. At times the debate has been quite contentious and polarized, but most workers today recognize the utility of both activities in specific situations—hence, the common term *consultation-liaison service.*

Psychosomatic medicine deals with mind-body and body-mind interactions in health and disease. Psychosomatic medicine is the basic science of the consultation-liaison psychiatrist or psychologist. *Pediatric psychiatry and psychology* represent expanded levels of activity in the pediatric setting. This area of child psychiatry and psychology is concerned with psychosocial issues associated with hospitalization, acute and chronic illness, somatic symptoms, stress response, psychosomatic disorder, and physical disability. The goal of a pediatric psychiatry service is to provide the full range of mental health services needed by these children and their families. In addition to consultation and liaison work, inpatient pediatric psychiatry units and various outpatient specialty clinics (e.g., pain clinic, enuresis clinic, and eating disorders clinic) are included.

B. HISTORICAL BACKGROUND

The child psychiatrist or psychologist who seeks to work in a pediatric environment should be aware of the developmental history of each discipline and the interactions of these disciplines to fully understand current attitudes and practice patterns. As reviewed by Richmond (1967), pediatrics became established in the 30 years between 1920 and 1950, which has been referred to as the "Golden Age of Curative Pediatrics." During this period, major advances in nutrition, intravenous therapy, immunizations, antibiotics, and hormone replacement (e.g., insulin) resulted in markedly decreased morbidity for children. Pediatricians established the controlled empirical investigation as the "gold standard" during this period, and they were absorbed in the purely organic sphere of illness. After World War II, urbanization, a burgeoning, increasingly mobile population, and the success of the new treatments in eliminating or controlling traditional pediatric illnesses led to many changes, but the expectation of cures and the organic emphasis continued as important residua of the Golden Age. In the past several decades, pediatrics has emphasized well-child care and shown increasing interest in behavioral and developmental problems, "the new morbidity" (Haggerty et al. 1975). The development of behavioral pediatrics as a subspecialty over the last 10 years is evidence of substantial pediatric investment in the psychological arena. However, this development is far from universally applauded by general and ambulatory pediatricians, many of whom see themselves in that role.

Child psychiatry evolved somewhat later than pediatrics and on an entirely separate track. In the 1920s, child psychiatry had its birth in child guidance clinics affiliated with the legal system. Medicine and psychiatry—and subsequently pediatrics and child psychiatry—were pushed together by an influential report in 1932 that decried the loss of humanistic values in an increasingly technologically based medical system, the overuse of laboratory tests with too little consideration of psychological disorders, and a deficient emphasis on prevention (Work 1989). To address these concerns, the report advocated integration of mental health disciplines into the hospital and an early version of the biopsychosocial model. Liaison programs and general hospital psychiatry services were developed to increase physicians' skills and improve patient care; the number of programs grew from 8 in 1932 to more than 1,000 today throughout the country. Pediatric psychiatry fellowships for pediatricians were established, and a small cadre of "retooled" pediatricians began to establish child psychiatric units within pediatrics, led by Leo Kanner at Johns Hopkins in 1930. Today, experience in the pediatric setting (via the consultation-liaison model) is a mandated component of child psychiatric training. However, satisfaction with the progress that has been made over the last 60 years must be tempered with the knowledge that 75% of child psychiatry programs allocate 10% or less of the total training time to the consultation-liaison experience (Fritz and Bergman 1984). As reflected by a number of scholarly articles (Anders 1977; Fritz 1990; Jellinek 1982), considerable work remains to be done before the child psychiatry–pediatrics relationship can be said to be truly collaborative. The interrelationships between the two evolutionary processes are summarized in Figure 1–1.

Developmental psychologists and pediatricians have collaborated on research in child development for many years, for example, in research concerning the effects of chronic illness on cognitive development. However, the delivery of clinical services by pediatric psychologists in hospital settings has evolved only within the last 25 years. In many hospital settings, psychologists

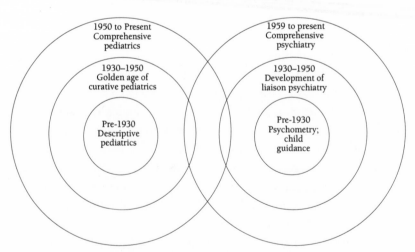

Figure 1–1.   Overlapping development of pediatrics and child psychiatry.

were initially seen merely as technicians who supplied psychometric data to the requesting physician. Over time, pediatric psychologists have become recognized as independent professionals with skills distinct from and complementing those of child psychiatrists. For example, on many consultation-liaison services, psychologists specialize in behavioral management programs and self-control training. Such interventions often significantly facilitate management of difficult patients and thus have come to be appreciated by nursing and medical staffs. The growth of pediatric psychology as a subspecialty in clinical psychology is reflected in the rapidly growing membership of the Society of Pediatric Psychology and the large number of high-quality, clinically relevant articles in the *Journal of Pediatric Psychology*. Nonetheless, the advances in pediatric psychology are much less known to practicing pediatricians than to mental health professionals.

C. THE HOSPITAL SYSTEM

A thorough understanding of the medical system—the institution, its values and expected etiquette, and the important players—is essential to be an effective consultant. The characteristics of the system, like an individual's personality traits, largely constitute a "given" for the consultant. Character change, in either an individual or a system, occurs only partially and in the course of a long and trusting relationship (assuming such change is even desired in the first place). To be effective, psychiatrists or psychologists consulting on a pediatric unit must recognize their outsider status and view themselves as resident aliens. They must acknowledge the realities of life in that foreign land, be familiar with the customs and cultural traditions, and speak the local dialect. At the same time, complete acceptance of the status quo means that the consultant cannot suggest changes and thus is destined to be ineffective. The consultant's close knowledge of the medical system results in recommendations that are maximally useful to the patient because they are likely to be implemented within the system.

1. Types of Hospitals

Hospitals differ by type (e.g., university, public, and private community) and even individual hospitals of the same type differ based on other variables. The type of hospital determines its basic mission and value structure. Virtually every hospital articulates its commitment to excellent patient care, but realistically, that commitment often coexists with other, sometimes competing priorities.

The *university hospital* values the training of physicians and the advancement of medical science to at least the same degree as patient care. Examples of this value system are readily identified. House staff rotate on a monthly basis for their own educational benefit; rarely is getting a new doctor in the middle of a hospitalization an advantage for the patient. A series of trainees interview and examine patients whether or not this is useful or comfortable for the patients. Faculty attending physicians rotate "off service" to their laboratories at arbitrary times and juggle academic pressures that pull against their commitment to patient care. The consultant who suggests a change in rotation schedule to ensure continuity of care for a patient or who recommends that the faculty attending physician rather than the resident perform the invasive procedures for a particular child is confronting the basic value system of a university hospital and faces an uphill battle.

The mission of *public hospitals* is to care for indigent patients. Economic problems, budget cutbacks, lack of options for ongoing care after discharge, the AIDS epidemic, rampant drug abuse, and a host of other depressing realities make this mission increasingly difficult to accomplish. The parents of children in a public hospital may have difficulty complying with the most basic treatment recommendations. The medical staff in most city and county hospitals in the United States are not ignorant of what constitutes comprehensive pediatric care. Rather, past experience and the enormity of the problems may result in a minimalist approach that overlooks options that may be feasible for a particular patient. The consultant in a public hospital who recommends an approach that is beyond the capacity of the pediatric unit to provide only engenders guilt and resentment in the staff and contributes nothing to the patient's care.

Private community hospitals serve the needs of practicing pediatricians and their patients. Typically, the resources of both the institution and the patients are greater than those found in either university or public hospitals. Private pediatricians have long-standing relationships with the families in their practices. They need and expect especially close communication about details of the consultant's evaluation as it proceeds. If a consultant makes suggestions directly to the patient or parents before discussing them thoroughly with the private pediatrician (even though such behavior would be appropriate or even expected in another type of hospital), the relationship is undercut and the consultant will see few referrals forthcoming. Financial issues (e.g., insurance coverage for consultation, the cost of mental health services, and who charges for what services) are more important in the community hospital than in a public institution, where such questions are often irrelevant for an individual patient.

2. System Characteristics

A number of real pressures may variably affect individual institutions of any type. If there is a shortage of available pediatric beds, the need to discharge patients as rapidly as possible to make room for new patients assumes great importance and usually makes the consultant's job more difficult. (Continuing an evaluation on an outpatient basis after initial contact is made in the hospital is one way to deal with the pressure.) When the average length of stay is 3–4 days, as it is on many pediatric wards, the staff's "mindset" is adjusted for very brief contact, and longer stays or evaluations are typically more difficult. In contrast, many empty beds constitute a financial burden, and the hospital will actively look for ways to fill them. In this situation, the staff as well as the consultant may have to grapple with issues of inappropriate admissions or pressures to prolong hospital stays. Low census may also present the consultant with the opportunity to do more definitive psychological interventions for specific patients that otherwise would not be possible within the pediatric setting.

The leadership, or lack of it, in the administration of a hospital is highly variable from one institution to another in terms of approachability, demonstrated interest in pediatrics, creativity in problem solving, efficiency in making the hospital run smoothly, and so forth. Even when available financial resources are equal, differences among hospitals' administrative philosophies and styles can result in vastly different experiences for both patients and staff, as illustrated by the following case example:

> In a large general hospital, the 90 pediatric beds constituted about 12% of the total. Dingy, substandard, and grossly outdated, the pediatric building was repeatedly slated for replacement and repeatedly "bumped" to a lower priority as adult facilities took precedence. The pediatric staff was demoralized and questioned the hospital's commitment to children. A new administration, in a worse financial climate, rapidly got new construction under way; morale soared among both patients and staff.
>
> Led by a long-term president who was nearing retirement, the hospital's administration seemed to be "on hold" for several years. Decisions were made with difficulty, the senior administrators were isolated and unavailable, and new ideas were met with little enthusiasm no matter what their merits were. A fatalistic, nothing-can-be-done attitude was pervasive on the wards. A new president infused energy, enthusiasm, and interest, with resulting changes evident at every level.

From the outset the consultant must be cognizant of the hospital leadership's characteristics and priorities, as they invariably filter down to affect aspects of patient care.

Children's hospitals also vary in their psychological sophistication in meeting the needs of hospitalized children and their families. A modern, progressive children's hospital has all of the following features routinely accessible for pediatric patients: 1) primary care nursing and continuity of care; 2) rooming-in for parents and a nearby medical inn (e.g., Ronald McDonald House); 3) family support services, including available pediatric social workers, parent advocates, and support and education groups; 4) a strong child life group providing recreational activities, therapeutic hospital play, and preoperative preparation; 5) an in-hospital school or tutors; and 6) a physical layout designed to reduce stress in waiting areas, provide for individual patient comfort, and allow parents and physicians to confer in privacy. When all these components are available, the consultant needs to be aware of them and encourage their appropriate use. When one or more of these components is lacking, the consultant must help staff creatively devise an approximation for particular patients while advocating for improvements within the institution. Examples of such creativity include obtaining the loan of a mobile home and permission to park it in the hospital lot when other nearby family lodging was not available, informally connecting experienced parents with those of a newly diagnosed child, and finding a skillful volunteer to help tutor and read to an immobilized child.

3. Previous Consultation

The new consultant to a pediatric unit must be aware of the unit's past experience with mental health consultation. If the history is an unhappy one, staff can be expected to view the new consultant skeptically, if not with rejection. Negative stereotypes of psychiatrists and psychologists abound in society, and medical professionals are far from immune to their influence. This fact, coupled with widespread ambivalence about involving mental health professionals in pediatric care, makes it easy for staff to focus on bad experiences, even if they were relatively rare. The new consultant should also recognize that mental health professionals' own prejudices, patronizing attitudes, or lack of expertise with pediatric patients are common and can contribute to a lukewarm welcome. A nondefensive, business-like approach followed by effective clinical work is the best path to success on a unit that has had prior negative experiences with consultation. Interestingly, the opposite situation, in which one replaces an effective, well-liked consultant, presents its own challenges. Filling the shoes of an established, respected, and familiar figure carries with it expectations and even resentments that are dealt with best when they are understood in context.

D. PROFESSIONAL STAFF ON A PEDIATRIC WARD

Important groups of professionals on a pediatric ward include physicians (attending and house staff), nurses, social workers, child life personnel, medical students, and secretaries. The professional identities distinguish staff by groups; within the groups, the characteristics of individual staff members are important.

1. Pediatricians

The attending pediatrician is at the top of the medical hierarchy, having final responsibility for the care of the patient. Often, the attending physician is the only staff member who has a long-term or continuing relationship with the patient. The developmental history of pediatrics as a discipline (described above), the selection process, and pediatric training together shape the image of the pediatrician in important ways. Although pediatricians are far from homogeneous, the consultant needs to be familiar with the characteristics of pediatricians and pediatric practice. These characteristics can be highlighted through a comparison with child psychiatry.

In an interesting series of projects, Enzer et al. (1986) examined the differences in views of childhood between pediatricians and child psychiatrists both before and after training. Pediatricians revealed an upbeat, optimistic attitude in which childhood was seen as happy, carefree, and pleasurable—the best time of life. Child psychiatrists saw childhood more as a time of struggle, powerlessness, and conflict. These attitudinal differences were present at the outset of training but increased afterward, suggesting that there is both a self-selection process among medical students and a reinforcement of different world views during training. Pediatricians' optimistic, positive orientation is associated with another important characteristic: the ability (and even need) to reassure effectively and decrease anxiety. Reassurance is a staple of pediatric practice, and often it constitutes a useful and efficient intervention. In contrast to child psychiatrists and psychologists, who must tolerate and sometimes provoke anxiety, pediatricians are less comfortable in dealing with anxiety and other strong emotion.

The practice of pediatrics is remarkably different from child psychiatry in a number of important ways. Historically, pediatricians have had a strong public health interest and have taken pride in helping large numbers of children. Pediatric practice is geared toward high volume and brief, though repeated interactions of 10–15 minutes. Child psychiatry, in contrast, has only recently embraced a public health orientation; typically, child psychiatry has a low-volume, long-interaction focus. It follows that pediatricians are extremely practical in their thinking about patients and oriented toward immediate concerns, whereas child psychiatrists are more reflective and theoretical, with a long-term orientation. In two respects, psychology is more akin to pediatrics than child psychiatry. First, the research of developmental psychologists working in pediatrics has often had greater implications for prevention than for direct clinical service. Second, the emergence of behavioral psychology as a primary orientation of most psychologists working in a consultation role in pediatrics has resulted in a focus on direct symptom management and brief, practical interventions that are congenial to the practice of pediatrics.

Pediatricians typically rely on parents, their own physical examinations of the child, and the laboratory to gather data; the child is frequently only a passive participant in the evaluation and treatment process. In contrast, the child psychiatry patient is usually an active contributor of diagnostic information and a central participant in psychotherapy. Pediatricians expect to treat all the children in a family, to acquire a good knowledge of and relationship with a family over time, and to see the children regularly, in times of health as well as illness. Child psychiatrists' and psychologists' contracts with families are usually more limited and tied to periods of maladjustment or psychopathology.

Unfortunately, the differences between the disciplines are often seen by one as deficiencies in the other, giving rise to prejudices that can doom effective collaboration. Summarizing an interview with an applicant for joint pediatric-psychiatric training, a faculty psychiatrist wrote, "She'll make an excellent psychiatrist; why would she waste her time in pediatrics?" A faculty pediatrician, rating a resident's performance in the same program, wrote, "He is nice, energetic, normal—it's unusual for such a person to be interested in psychiatry." Although pediatricians' attitudes are only indirectly approachable by individuals outside of pediatrics, psychiatrists and psychologists in the consultant role need to have dealt with any prejudices of their own at the outset. Differences need to be recognized and respected—not to be seen as shortcomings. Consultants should not seek to remake pediatricians in their own image. They can, however, take comfort in the fact that pediatricians' views of mental health professionals vary with age: research shows that younger pediatricians, whose training took place after the increasing emphasis on behavioral pediatrics, are more likely to involve psychiatrists and psychologists with their patients smoothly and frequently (Fritz and Bergman 1985).

2. House Staff

Although the characteristics of pediatric practice are relevant to all pediatricians, house staff have a unique set of issues that are relevant to the mental health consultant. Pediatric residents are in the process of forming their professional identity during a period of intense learning. Basic technical aspects of pediatrics, such as procedures, fluid management, and obtaining appropriate laboratory results, have not yet become second nature for junior residents and frequently take precedence over less tangible and immediate problems involving the consultant. Residents rarely have sufficient time on a given rotation to become thoroughly comfortable in their roles and level of competence. Their frontline position gives them a perspective that may differ significantly from the attending pediatrician's, with associated potential for confusion and conflict. Long, stressful hours and sleep deprivation may compromise a house officer's patience and objectivity. Being free of a difficult patient, pleasing an attending physician, or getting off duty may become primary values for a stressed resident. The experienced consultant will consider the unique issues that house officers bring to patient care and find a middle ground between accepting or defending the status quo and suggesting impossible solutions.

Bearing in mind the general nature of pediatrics will clearly be helpful to the consultant, but it does not substitute for personal contact with individual physicians when beginning as a consultant to a pediatric ward. The unit director, subspecialist heads, and chief resident are important individuals to introduce oneself to either formally or over coffee. The consultant should determine how knowledgeable and interested these individuals are in the psychosocial aspects of care. Opinions, beliefs, and past experiences regarding psychiatrists and psychologists should be sought. Any reservations about the consultant's age, gender, pediatric experience, availability, and so forth are better discussed immediately rather than after they produce conflict. Expectations regarding use of psychoactive medications, behavioral regimens, or the consultant's directly writing orders or taking over aspects of care need to be clarified with individual physicians to avoid subsequent confusion. The financial realities and billing procedures should also be discussed.

3. Nurses

Nurses constitute the largest group of professionals on the pediatric ward, and their role places them in the most frequent direct contact with the patient. Nursing training also emphasizes humanistic aspects of care to a greater degree than does physician training. For these reasons, nurses are directly or indirectly responsible for a significant proportion of consultation requests. The history of nurse-physician professional relationships has not been a smooth one over the years, and interdisciplinary communication problems continue to complicate the provision of care in hospitals. Florence Nightingale, the founder of nursing as a profession, exerted her considerable influence largely by convincing powerful male physicians and politicians to promote her revolutionary ideas while she maintained her position as a weak, feeble woman confined to a sick bed for over 50 years. Hospital training schools for nurses, which she pioneered, emphasized service, long hours, and submissive behavior rather than education. The belief that a physician was always right— and that even when he was wrong he must be made to appear right—was long a cornerstone of nurses' training (Kalisch and Kalisch 1977).

The community college movement, a growing shortage of nurses, more women in medicine, and consciousness-raising associated with the women's movement have brought about significant changes within nursing. Administrative shifts in hospitals have given nurses increased autonomy—at least on paper. However, physicians at all levels of training, in addition to the nursing hierarchy, give "orders" to staff nurses. Nurses still are frequently deferential to physicians, a deference maintained by sociologic factors, such as the preponderance of women in nursing compared to men, the lower average socioeconomic status of nurses, and the disparity in educational levels. When nurses resent physicians' patronizing attitudes and lack of respect, they may adopt a passive-aggressive posture that invariably undermines patient care.

The consultant must know how and to what degree the evolution of nursing has proceeded in the specific hospital. Within a given nursing staff, it is likely that some individuals will have retained rather traditional beliefs about a nurse's role, whereas others will be more progressive and assertive. It is essential to recognize that the nurses usually have a wealth of information about patients gleaned from the intimate contact associated with bedside care. This information may or may not be volunteered; if it is not, the consultant should actively solicit it and subsequently be especially attuned to physician-nurse communication in other areas. The consultant must also be familiar with nurses' workloads, rotation schedules, and the like to be sure that recommendations have a possibility of being implemented. For example, it is pointless to recommend the continuity of a primary care nurse when registry nurses provide much of the care on a ward, or to request that nurses carry out a contingent reinforcement plan when the staffing level will not permit sufficient nursing time to be devoted to it.

4. Social Workers

In many children's hospitals, the pediatric social worker has been the frontline mental health professional, although pediatric social workers typically have not been formal members of the consultation-liaison service. In the past 5 years, largely as a consequence of tightening medical economics, social work departments have suffered cutbacks that reduce their capacity to provide services at previous levels. Responses to these cutbacks have varied. In some institutions, routine contact with a social worker is not provided, and social workers respond to consultation requests according to a set of guidelines. In others, only the most basic and concrete services are provided, such as obtaining insurance or welfare coverage, arranging dispositions, and so forth. In some hospitals, the availability of social workers varies even from one service or ward to another. The child psychiatrist or psychologist must be familiar with social service resources in his or her particular institution and establish a working relationship with the individual social workers who cover the pediatric unit. Without such "homework," the consultant risks at least redundancy and lack of coordination in efforts and, at worst, turf battles that drain everyone's energy. Roles and duties cannot be expected to be the same across institutions, but they must be clarified for the consultees on the unit, as well as for the consultant and the social worker who will frequently be involved in many of the same cases. Although the roles of consultant psychiatrist, psychologist, and social worker can overlap and, with communication and creativity, be varied from case to case, the social worker's unique familiarity with community resources should be recognized. Access to home health care programs, visiting nurse associations, self-help and medical education groups, and various charitable agencies can rarely be duplicated by other mental health professionals.

5. Child Life Workers

Child life workers are a unique group of professionals who have no counterparts in the adult sections of the hospital. Their job is to normalize the hospital environment so that children and their parents can continue to function and develop despite the stresses of hospitalization. They maintain areas of a ward that are limited to play and age-appropriate recreational activities. Group meetings and projects, preparation for medical procedures, prevention work, and individualized programs can be developed by child life specialists, who frequently have an abundance of energy and ideas. Because the child life group does not bill separately for services and does not provide direct medical intervention, their influence and stature in the power hierarchy of a hospital are often tenuous. The consultant is well advised to involve child life workers in both the evaluation and the treatment phases of consultation. Sometimes the consultant can effectively underline and emphasize the recommendations that have already been made by the child life workers but gone unheeded.

5. Other Staff Members

There are two other groups in a pediatric hospital who are often ignored by the consultant psychiatrist or psychologist, usually to the consultant's detriment. The unit secretary manages the schedules of the patients, organizes the paperwork, and knows almost everyone in the hospital. The secretary is a very important person, especially if she or he has been working on the unit for a significant period of time. The consultant who does not have such an established, central figure as an ally will find that notes get lost, records are unavailable, and the patient is off the ward at inopportune times. A polite introduction and a friendly relationship with the unit secretary will lead to good advice as to how and when things really get done on that unit. The second group who are easily but unwisely overlooked are medical students. Although they are transient and inexperienced, medical students may get extremely involved and form important relationships with individual patients. Their observations and history obtained from a patient may be more detailed and insightful than the information available from more senior members of the medical team. If the patient is "difficult" for one reason or another, others may tacitly abandon aspects of the care to the medical student as the lowest person on the medical ladder.

Awareness of the nature of the system in which one will be working and of the characteristics of the practice of pediatrics helps the consultant approach the system with appropriate expectations. Discussions with individuals who will use the consultation service help them to know what to expect as well. The stage is thus set for the interaction to be clinically useful and professionally satisfying.

E. REFERENCES

Anders TF: Child psychiatry and pediatrics: the state of the relationship. Pediatrics 60:616–620, 1977

Caplan G: The Theory and Practice of Mental Health Consultation. New York, Basic Books, 1970

Enzer NB, Singleton DS, Snellman LA, et al: Interferences in collaboration between child psychiatrists and pediatricians: a fundamental difference in attitude toward childhood. Journal of Developmental and Behavioral Pediatrics 7:186–193, 1986

Fritz GK: Consultation-liaison in child psychiatry and the evolution of pediatric psychiatry. Psychosomatics 31:85–90, 1990

Fritz GK, Bergman AS: Consultation-liaison training for child psychiatrists: results of a survey. Gen Hosp Psychiatry 6:25–29, 1984

Fritz GK, Bergman AS: Child psychiatrists seen through pediatricians' eyes: results of a national survey. J Am Acad Child Psychiatry 24:81–86, 1985

Haggerty RJ, Roghmann KJ, Pleses IB: Child Health and the Community. New York, Wiley, 1975

Jellinek MS: The present status of child psychiatry in pediatrics. N Engl J Med 1227–1230, 1982

Kalisch BJ, Kalisch PA: An analysis of the sources of physician-nurse conflict. J Nurs Adm 7:50–57, 1977

Richmond JB: Child development: a basic science for pediatrics. Pediatrics 39:649–658, 1967

Work H: The "menace of psychiatry" revisited: the evolving relationship between pediatrics and child psychiatry. Psychosomatics 30:86–93, 1989

CHAPTER TWO

The Process of Consultation on a Pediatric Unit

Gregory K. Fritz, M.D.
Anthony Spirito, Ph.D.

T he background work has been completed, the psychiatrist or psychologist is sufficiently knowledgeable about the hospital environment, and he or she is familiar with the needs and characteristics of the staff working on the pediatric unit. Now, he or she is ready to begin the actual work of consulting. This chapter provides a concrete, step-by-step description of how one does a consultation on a pediatric ward, while recognizing that a "cookbook" plan has limitations and that the individual child, family, and clinical situation usually require flexibility in approach. This chapter is organized chronologically, from the intake to the writing of the consultation note. A detailed discussion of problems commonly encountered is presented in Chapter 3, and a description of interventions available to the consultant follows in Chapter 4.

A. INTAKE

The first contact a member of the pediatric staff has with the consultant is through the intake process, in which a consultation is requested for a particular patient. The intake sets the tone for all that is to follow, for both the consultee and the consultant. Thus, the intake process deserves enough thought and refinement to make it smooth, reliable, and businesslike. Psychiatrists or psychologists joining an established service should make sure they themselves understand the intake process and that it makes sense. If it does not, or if the service is being newly organized, the way in which a consultation request is received should be spelled out specifically. Typically, a secretary responds to a telephone request and elicits basic information that allows the consultation to proceed. The request is carefully logged, a simple procedure but one that allows accurate troubleshooting should a problem develop (pertaining, for example, to the speed of the response or who initiated the consultation). The intake log also provides a ready mechanism for reviewing the progress and growth of the consultation service. The intake information obtained and recorded on a prepared consultation form should include 1) the patient's name, birth date, and location in the hospital; 2) the name of the physician requesting the consultation and the phone or beeper number; 3) the presenting problem or reason for the request; 4) the level of urgency; and 5) insurance information.

The secretary who does the intake needs to have good communication skills, thorough training in the workings of the service and the requirements of the intake process, and ready access to the director of the service in case unforeseen questions arise. Individuals new to the consultation service should be personally introduced to the intake process by this secretary. Because the pediatric unit can feel like unfamiliar territory to a psychiatrist or psychologist, every bit of concrete information that can be provided for a new consultant is helpful. Table 2–1 summarizes additional, relevant orientation information that a consultant should have in a readily available form before beginning the clinical work.

A critical point to be determined at intake is whether the consultation request is routine or emergent. Emergency consultations need a response within the hour, and every service must have a mechanism for providing such a response. We have found that the most useful definition of what constitutes an emergency is "whatever the referring physician says is an emergency, when asked directly." This rather inclusive definition carries with it the possibility that the consultant will rush to find a situation that was emergent only in terms of the consultee's anxiety. In these rather infrequent circumstances, the worst that happens is that the service is seen to respond more rapidly than necessary—a perception that is never harmful. The use of this definition avoids dickering about details or giving the impression that the service is unavailable. A number of years' experience with this procedure has shown that it is rarely abused.

Patients for whom nonemergent consultations are requested are seen within 24 hours, but the "earlier equals better" rule applies to the consultation process in both directions: the earlier in a patient's hospitalization a consultation is requested, and the earlier the consultant responds to the request, the better. Corridor discussions represent a legitimate method for receiving consultation requests, but such information needs to be channeled into the regular intake process for subsequent problems to be avoided.

Everyone involved with the consultation service should be aware of populations that are and are not eligible for service. Commonly, a child psychiatric consultation service will see 1) patients 18 years of age or younger and 2) any patient hospitalized on the pediatric service

Table 2–1.   Orientation: relevant information a new consultant should establish or obtain

1. Succinct statement of how consultees request consultation: eligibility, phone number to call, procedure, hours of service, response time, emergency procedure
2. Names of heads of units, services, or specialty groups—and their areas of responsibilities—for whom consultations will be provided
3. Map of relevant areas of the institution
4. Legal procedures particular to the state and institution re
    a. Involuntary commitment
    b. Use of restraints
    c. Use of 1:1 "sitters"
    d. Security guards—use and availability
    e. Discharge against medical advice
5. Billing practices for consultation

(to include older individuals treated by pediatricians, such as those with cystic fibrosis or developmental disabilities). A succinct statement of eligibility requirements and intake procedures should be printed up and distributed to the pediatric units, staff, and attending pediatricians, as well as to each of the psychiatrists and psychologists who will be providing consultation services.

B. PREINTERVIEW STEPS

1. Determining the Reason for Referral

Although an effort is made to determine the reason for the consultation request at the time of intake, experienced consultants know that this information is incomplete or inaccurate much of the time. The referring physician may not even be aware that there are interpersonal problems between the patient and staff or that the patient has an underlying psychiatric disorder or major stresses that determine the need for consultation. Alternately, the physician may be aware of his or her own negative feelings toward the patient, personal overinvolvement, or impending vacation but may be unwilling to explicitly present the difficult issue as the central problem. In the extreme, some physicians seem to believe "if a patient or parent doesn't like me, they must be crazy," but this is rarely written as the reason for requesting consultation. The following case example illustrates how the stated and actual reasons for the consultation can be discrepant:

> Psychiatric consultation was sought by a plastic surgeon treating a 4-year-old boy for trauma to his foot; the request stated "pain control, behavior problem." In discussing the case with the consultant, the surgeon revealed his thinly veiled disgust with the boy's parents: they were "demanding," "intrusive," and "inappropriate." During the evaluation, the parents voiced dissatisfaction with the surgeon's infrequent, unpredictable visits; superficial responses to their questions; and dismissal of what they perceived

as their son's extreme pain. They feared they'd made a bad choice of physicians and that their son would suffer; their anxiety and guilt fueled the boy's discomfort and negative behavior. The consultant worked to help the surgeon meet the parents' needs for intellectual understanding and a sense of some control. A succinct summary of the dynamic issues, an explanation of the parents' educational backgrounds, and a very clear prescription of how management needed to be modified for the case to go better proved helpful in this regard.

In short, it is crucial to begin the consultation by speaking with the referring physician to discover, clarify, or reaffirm the purpose of the consultation. In this discussion, one must both register the explicit concerns that the physician has regarding the patient and listen for unspoken issues that may be equally or more important; both need to be addressed in the consultation work.

At times, especially in university hospitals, the referring physician, the attending physician of record, and the primary physician who knows the patient best may not be the same individual. In such a case, the consultant must use his or her judgment in determining whom to contact, guided by the rule that it never hurts to talk to any physician involved in the case. Sometimes, even the diligent consultant cannot find out who in practical terms has active responsibility for the patient's care. Nobody may. Such circumstances often involve "care by committee," in which subspecialist consultants direct the portions of care that fall into their particular area of expertise, as illustrated in the following case example:

A 15-year-old girl with short gut syndrome had been maintained all her life on total parenteral nutrition (TPN). Psychiatric consultation was requested because both she and her family were seen as resistant to the prospect of beginning eating. During the evaluation, it became clear that two surgeons, the pediatric gastroenterologist, her private pediatrician, the hospital TPN team, a dietitian, and a pharmacist who for years had prepared the TPN supplements all had direct input to the family and advocated multiple, conflicting plans from their own perspective. The lack of agreement and leadership fueled the patient's and family's anxiety about changing a lifelong, lifesaving procedure. The consultant organized several case conferences, the outcome of which was to define a single attending physician and a protocol for gradual introduction of oral food.

Recognition that an unfortunate leadership arrangement is operating constitutes an important systems diagnosis that is always relevant to patient care.

2. Preparation of the Patient and Family

In addition to the reason for the consultation, it is important to ascertain how the patient and parents have been prepared for the psychiatrist's or psychologist's visit. One cannot assume that the family has been notified of the impending consultation or that the preparation was appropriate or useful. It is disconcerting to encounter a patient who is not expecting you. Even worse is the parent who believes a mental health consultation means that the primary physician "thinks my child is crazy" or "has given up and wants to get rid of us." An experienced consultant advises the referring physician, gently and early, on how to prepare the family for consultation. Ideally, the pediatrician describes to both the patient and the family his or her desire to "leave no stone unturned" in his ongoing efforts to be effective in managing the clinical problem. Consultation is presented as an adjunct to treatment; the patient and family are explicitly reassured of the pediatrician's continued primary role. Describing the consultation as a common or routine feature of the medical management of the disorder may alleviate some of the stigma that may be associated with the decision to consult a psychiatrist or psychologist. The pediatrician's straightforward presentation of the purpose of the consultation, a firm belief in the desirability of mental health involvement, and when possible, personal familiarity with the individual consultant will usually make the psychological evaluation acceptable.

3. Further Preliminary Steps

In addition to the referring physician, the consultant should discuss with other knowledgeable staff their perceptions of the patient's problems. Commonly, the primary care nurse has a wealth of information about the patient based on bedside observations. Other professionals may also have useful information to share, including the social worker, chief resident, child life worker, medical student, chaplain, or—especially when a language other than English is spoken—any hospital staff member who has had significant contact with the patient or family. Because of confidentiality issues, one must be cautious of speaking with visitors, particularly peers of the patient, even if they seem eager to offer their help. In general, it is better to speak only with professional staff before having direct contact with the parents or the patient.

It is worthwhile to review the medical record early on in a consultation. This review should include the admission workup, progress notes, other consultants' reports, and laboratory data for the present admission, as well as the old records from past admissions. Previous psychosocial consultation notes are especially useful, as they provide a baseline against which to compare current functioning. If nursing notes are not part of the progress notes, they should be located in their separate section, for they are an invaluable source of data, as the following case example illustrates:

A 6-year-old boy recovering from trauma sustained in a car accident was extremely anxious around physical therapy, dressing changes, and procedures. Hospital play, individual sessions, and rewards for cooperative behavior were minimally helpful, puzzling the medical staff and the consultant. The nursing notes summarized a late night conversation between the mother and a nurses' aide, in which the mother expressed many fears about her child's prognosis and a serious misunderstanding of the extent of the injuries and the prognosis. Clarification of these issues allayed her anxieties, and her son rapidly became more relaxed and cooperative.

Child psychiatric consultants should not dismiss their medical knowledge as they review the chart; it is legitimate and often helpful to rethink the diagnostic workup and the treatment plan. Psychologists as well should apply their common sense and medical experience when reviewing the medical record. If concerned about possible interactions or side effects of medications in the patient's regimen, the psychologist should not hesitate to discuss the case with a psychiatric colleague.

C. PARENT INTERVIEW

The first direct contact is usually made with the parents. A sick child's parents want to maintain their decision-making and protective roles (although the hospital environment challenges these roles with the addition of multiple, variably intrusive authority figures). Preferably, a physician or nurse who knows and is trusted by the family introduces the consultant to the parents. The parents thus have the opportunity to meet the consultant, share their concerns, and bring up questions or misunderstandings they may harbor. Introduction by a staff member also helps the consultant avoid embarrassing miscues and confusion, such as the one illustrated in the following case example:

> A resident child psychiatrist, after a brief discussion with staff at the nursing station, went to see John Smith, a 13-year-old boy with recurrent abdominal pain. Entering a two-patient room, he saw a young teenager sitting with his parents. "I'm Dr. Young. I meet many of the patients on the gastroenterology service, and Dr. Jones asked me to consult with you. You must be John." The boy nodded, and he and his parents began an animated conversation with the psychiatrist. Only after an hour had passed, extensive history about the family, adolescent development, and so forth had been obtained, and the psychiatrist had begun to schedule a subsequent meeting did it become clear that he had consulted on the wrong case. The intended patient, a roommate also named John who was hospitalized with the same symptoms, had gone to radiology. (The Smiths, initially puzzled, had found the discussion interesting.)

A detailed history of the child's illness may or may not be obtained from the parents at the time of the introduction. Because a psychological evaluation takes a significant block of time, extended interviews with either the parents or the child should be scheduled in advance with the ward secretary. Such an arrangement gives parents a feeling of predictability and structure, and it ensures that the consultant will not arrive on the ward to find the parents gone from the hospital or the patient off the unit. Perhaps because the seriousness of a hospitalization changes everyone's schedule, fathers are frequently as available as mothers; the consultant often finds it easier to interview both parents together on a pediatric ward than in an outpatient clinic. In any case, the expectation that both parents will participate should be set forth and adhered to insofar as possible.

D. EVALUATION OF THE CHILD

In general, as with any psychological evaluation, the child should be seen individually as a routine part of the consultation. Occasionally, parental questions or difficulties will be the sole reason for the consultation, or a young child will be unwilling to separate from parents under the stress of hospitalization. In such cases, the consultant should forgo a separate evaluation of the child, at least for the moment, and proceed as clinical judgment dictates. Usually, however, the consultant needs to arrange for a private, nonregressed setting in which to see the child. This means that a private office or playroom is preferable to a ward room, out of bed or sitting up is preferable to lying down, dressed or modestly covered is preferable to being exposed, and so forth. Creativity and flexibility in this regard are required on most pediatric wards, but one should not compromise beyond what is clinically reasonable. Just because a child is hospitalized does not mean it is easier or more appropriate to talk about personal topics with roommates looking on and nurses bustling in and out. The consultant who views a psychological evaluation as a very important undertaking worthy of significant logistical rearrangement communicates a serious sense of purpose to the staff, the family, and the patient.

1. Building an Alliance

A psychological evaluation of a child entails the establishment of an alliance between the child and the psychiatrist or psychologist, and a consultation on a pediatric ward is no exception. The first step is to consider whether the child is as comfortable as possible; bedpans, intravenous equipment, positioning, and pain medication may need attention. The consultant's sensitivity in this regard is usually appreciated. The consultant must clarify his or her mission, relating it to something the child notices and can acknowledge. The consultant must be clear about not knowing the outcome before the evaluation is carried out: "The doctors and nurses working with you told me you're having a hard time remembering your insulin and that the shots hurt a lot. Sometimes I'm able to help kids with those sorts of problems. Let's talk together a couple of times, get to know each other and then decide if there are things we can do to make it go better." For younger children, a doctor's bag of carefully selected toys (e.g., medical equipment, a family of dolls, a deck of cards for interactive play, magic markers and paper, small animals and cars, a toy telephone, a space gun to express aggression) is a needed icebreaker. The following case example illustrates the importance of a consultant's toys in establishing an alliance with a younger child:

> A 7-year-old girl with multiple surgical complications after a bladder repair was referred because she was oppositional and withdrawn, and the question of medication had been raised. At the initial contact with the consultant, she turned in bed toward the wall and refused to talk. Returning later with a bag of toys, the consultant engaged the child with a display of syringes, intravenous equipment, splints, and a stethoscope. The child vengefully gave injections to the consultant, immobilized a doll, and prescribed painful procedures that conveyed her anger at what she experienced as undeserved punishment. The consultant returned with his bag of toys on a daily basis, and each time the child plunged into enthusiastic, aggressive play around the medical theme. In the course of the sessions, the consultant clar-

ified the nonpunitive nature of the surgery, provided factual information at the child's level, and encouraged ventilation of feelings. The child, although far from docile, became more cooperative with treatment and easier to involve in ward activities.

2. The Interview

The consultant should address the issues that provoked the referral, but the timing and format of the evaluation are individually determined. Despite the immediacy of the hospitalization and the medical problem, the consultant should make clear that he or she is interested in the whole child. Recognition that the child is a student, a sibling, a team member, and a friend as well as a patient should be conveyed. The child's strengths, interests, preferences, and life outside the hospital should be explored. Frequently the medical team lacks the time or the focus to get details about the nonmedical aspects of a child's life, and obtaining this information helps shed light on a variety of in-hospital problems, as illustrated by the following case example:

> A young teenager with diabetes was referred for noncompliance with his regimen. Initially surly and sarcastic, he warmed up gradually in response to questions about his athletic interests, school activities, and pet snake. It became clear that his noncompliance was largely around his dietary restrictions; although secretive, he was conscientious about his urine testing and insulin administration. He ate "junk food" with his peers because he was afraid they'd think he was sickly or weird if he didn't. Understanding these issues and the limited extent of the noncompliance helped the staff feel more positively toward him, and he responded favorably (although he continued his dietary indiscretions).

The evaluation should also include an assessment of the child's cognitive understanding of the illness—its cause, symptoms, treatment, and prognosis—and associated fears and expectations. A direct inquiry about how young patients would like themselves or their family to change can elicit a basis for subsequent interventions.

3. Mental Status and Physical Examination

A mental status examination should always be a part of a mental health consultation. The elements of the mental status examination can be elicited in a formal series of questions or inserted in the interview at opportune times, but a concise, baseline description of mental functioning is always useful. When changing levels of consciousness, fluctuating mood, or impaired thought processes are an issue, serial mental status examinations are indicated. Ward staff are often unable to articulate what they have observed about the patient's mental functioning, especially with younger children; the consultant's mental status description serves as a useful model.

For child psychiatrists, the question of whether to do all or part of a physical examination as part of a consultation is best decided on an individual basis. Although a physical examination is seldom a part of an outpatient psychiatric evaluation, it fits more easily with the expectations of a patient on a pediatric ward. Some patients benefit psychologically from the consultant physically examining an area of the body that has been injured or affected by illness or treatment; they may respond to the consultant's empathy or may be helped to confront reality. Although few psychiatrists pride themselves on the acuity of their current skills in physical diagnosis, most who have examined patients in the course of consultation have at one time or another made important, unexpected discoveries, as the following case example illustrates:

> A child psychiatrist was asked to consult on a patient who appeared to the house staff to be suffering from obvious anorexia nervosa. The 15-year-old girl presented with significant weight loss that she described as desired, peculiar eating habits, amenorrhea, and a perfectionist, controlling personality that made her a management problem. Concluding her evaluation with a physical examination, the consultant found papilledema that had been overlooked because the staff had jumped to a premature conclusion. The workup was subsequently intensified at the consultant's urging, and a craniopharyngioma was ultimately discovered.

Generally, the psychiatrist's major contribution to the patient's management will not come from repeating others' physical examinations. Sometimes, being in the unique position of not examining the child allows a consultant access to information not available to those who must probe and disturb.

E. OTHER INFORMATION

Standardized assessment instruments are generally underused by pediatric consultants. Self-report questionnaires, parental report measures, and observer rating scales have been developed for specific pediatric populations. The consultant who administers them routinely as part of an evaluation taps an important source of data and gets a quantitative summary of relevant symptoms or behaviors. Selected scales that are appropriate for use with particular pediatric patients are described and referenced in Appendix 2–1.

Several issues that are commonplace in outpatient mental health evaluations are no less important in pediatric consultation. The need for outside information, beyond what the parents and child can provide, may present a problem. A child's school teacher, caseworker, probation officer, or therapist may have important information that will help in interpreting particular changes. Information concerning a child's intelligence, language ability, or academic achievement may be available from external sources. The consultant should not be resigned to doing without crucial information just because it is not at hand and time is short. By using the authority of the children's hospital and a degree of urgency, and with the parent giving a phone release, the consultant can rapidly obtain important information from outside sources.

F. CONFIDENTIALITY

The issue of confidentiality, never a simple one when dealing with children or adolescents and their parents, is more complicated in consultation work. The consultant becomes involved in the case at the request of the attending physician and it is assumed that the consultant will provide the expert opinion at least to that individual. The consultation report will become part of the medical record and, as such, available to every professional on the ward. These facts should be made clear to both the parents and the child at the outset. At the same time, the consultant's clinical judgment allows the determination of what information is and is not useful to the primary physician and the ward staff. If the child or the parents provide information that is not relevant to the pediatrician's care of the child and request that it be kept confidential, the consultant is justified in doing so. Such a request is made relatively infrequently, and care must be taken not to be backed into an untenable position where the data behind the consultant's recommendations cannot be shared with the staff.

G. INITIAL RECOMMENDATIONS

After the initial evaluation, the psychiatrist or psychologist should again make contact with the staff before leaving the unit. The purposes of this discussion are 1) to share the initial impression and the plan to complete the consultation and 2) to deal with any urgent concerns the consultant or the staff may have. Such concerns include a deteriorating medical condition as identified by the consultant, suicidal or self-destructive behavior in the child, behavior that is dangerous to the ward and needs immediate management, the risk of elopement or the parents signing the child out against medical advice, or significant anger or anxiety on the part of the staff that needs to be addressed at once. The fast pace of an acute pediatric unit does not always allow the consultant to defer management advice until a thorough evaluation is accomplished. However, most of the issues of urgent concern to a pediatric staff are fairly gross, and the experienced consultant can respond to them effectively despite limited information. Familiarity with legal procedures that are applicable to urgent situations in one's own state and institution is essential for an efficient response (as noted in Table 2–1).

Some psychiatrists and psychologists, confronted with a staff eager for their wisdom, are tempted to "shoot from the hip" and provide extensive formulations and recommendations based on extremely scanty information. This temptation should be resisted because one's long-range accuracy in such situations tends to be poor.

H. CONSULTATION REPORT

The formal summary of the consultant's opinion on a case is contained in the written consultation report. Although notes in the medical chart should not be expected to replace personal communication with pediatric staff, they are an essential, permanent record of the work done and the conclusions reached. A cardinal rule of pediatric consultation is always to leave a note. Even when one is in the midst of an evaluation and not in a position to write the definitive report, a short note of the work in progress should be made at every visit to the unit. A note such as "Consultation under way to evaluate noncompliance; patient interviewed, meeting with parents tomorrow at 10 A.M.; report to follow" is brief but extremely helpful to others involved in the child's care. Such notes have become increasingly important for billing and medicolegal purposes as well.

Psychiatrists and psychologists tend to value comprehensiveness, rich supporting data, subtle detail, and thoroughness in case reports prepared in outpatient clinics or inpatient psychiatric units. Preparation of such reports may consist largely of organizing a mountain of information that has been obtained, with relatively little detail omitted in the final document. An eight-page summary that begins in utero and includes an exhaustive description of every aspect of the child's and family's current life may be useful in a psychiatric setting, but it is inappropriate as a consultation report, for two major reasons. First, it is so long that it will not be read; unread, it will contribute nothing to the patient's care. For this reason, most consultants limit their written reports to one or two pages. Second, an eight-page report almost certainly contains personal details that are inappropriate and unnecessary in a medical chart that is open to a wide and often unsophisticated readership. Brevity helps assure appropriate confidentiality.

The challenge for a psychiatrist or psychologist in writing a consultation report is to be succinct, understandable, and practical without oversimplifying a complex clinical problem. The format for a consultation report follows the medical model: 1) identifying information/reason for consultation; 2) history—of the present problem, past development, and family; 3) mental status examination; 4) diagnosis and formulation; and 5) recommendations. Although other formats might work as well, the medical schema ensures consistency across consultants and is familiar to the physicians and nurses who will use the report.

The *reason for the consultation* is a distillation of the overt request received at intake and the clarification or amplification obtained from discussions with staff. It is usually an improvement on both and may serve to focus the staff's perception of the patient's problems. This statement also sets forth the consultant's orientation to the evaluation and the information that follows. The *history* section is kept brief by not repeating historical material that is already in the chart. A consultation note should include only salient additional history and corrections of misinformation. Summary statements are used rather than detailed examples that illustrate or prove an historical point. "Academic failure, delinquency and drug use" efficiently summarizes a great deal of history that would be described in much greater detail in an inpatient psychiatric workup; such a summary is appropriate in a consultation report. Results of the *mental status examination* are reported succinctly, with more detail supplied when there are abnormal findings. The cross-sectional nature of the mental status examination is both its strength and its weakness, and the note should reflect the situation, timing, and so forth of the examination. Suicidality is an important factor in many consultations, and documentation of a patient's suicide potential is especially important. A DSM-III-R (American Psychiatric Association 1987) *diagnosis* is generally of more interest to mental health professionals than the pediatric staff, who usually desire help rather than labels. Nevertheless, a diagnosis is included in the logical progression of a psychological evaluation. It is useful descriptively and often makes billing easier as well. On many pediatric consultation services, the most common diagnostic codes are adjustment reactions (code 309) and psychological factors associated with diseases classified elsewhere (code 316); thus, further clarification is obviously necessary. A clearly worded *formulation* conveys the essence of the consultant's opinion and paves the way for the recommendations that follow. The following case examples, taken directly from consultation reports, illustrate, first, a useful formulation and, then, two formulations that are variously flawed:

> Regarding a 15-year-old referred for poor compliance with his cystic fibrosis treatment: "Patient is a highly intelligent, well-motivated young man whose denial (the basis for poor compliance) has served him well in many respects but who now needs to confront and embrace his cystic fibrosis to fight it effectively. He uses intellectual defenses well and these need to be supported while emotional issues (fear, sadness, resentment, etc.) are actively identified and discussed. Supportive family is a major resource."
>
> Regarding a 14-year-old girl with recurrent abdominal pain: "She has a wish for life as it existed around the turn of the century and cultivates her tomboyish 'Tom Sawyer' personality. She has some of these ideas secondary to her mother's earlier life (mother didn't have to go to school much) which seems idealized. Her mother idealizes Susan's maternal grandmother and great aunt as 'perfect women.' This great aunt died of appendicitis when she was 14 (Susan's age) and Susan's mother was 7—an early morning incident that still upsets Susan's mother. Susan says she is like this aunt (artistically) who was taken 'by God' because she was too perfect. It seems that she is quite concerned that her stomach pains and discomforts may mean that she will be taken 'by God.' She indeed tries not to be angry and to be 'perfect' like this great aunt. This script has not been entirely conscious to her and probably not to the mother but may well be operating in this family."
>
> Regarding a 12-year-old boy with ulcerative colitis who had behavior problems and an observed difficult relationship with his mother: "Suspect depression with dysfunctional family."

The *recommendation* section of the report is the most closely read component. As such, it should not be squeezed into the last two lines of the consultation form or dashed off hurriedly under the mistaken impression that interventions follow obviously from the formulation.

The recommendations should be organized in terms of priority—further evaluation that needs to take place, psychopharmacologic or behavioral management that should be implemented promptly, plans for the rest of the hospitalization, and long-term recommendations. The details of how and by whom the interventions should be carried out should be concretely specified. Finally, the report is concluded with the consultant's legible name and signature and a telephone extension where he or she can be reached should questions or problems arise before the follow-up visit, which is also specified.

I. SUMMARY

Some consultants are clearly more successful than others in working within pediatrics. A broadly useful knowledge base, an interest in the area, and good interpersonal skills are necessary but not sufficient characteristics of the consultant whose input will be valued and sought on subsequent cases. Familiarity with the consultation process as described in this chapter and the previous chapter will greatly enhance one's effectiveness. Table 2–2 summarizes the es-

Table 2–2.   "Ten Commandments" of consultation-liaison work

1. Know the realities of life in the system within which you are consulting.
2. Expect the first referrals to be difficult "test" cases, and work hard.
3. Be available; a consultation-liaison service should be prompt and user-friendly in taking consultation requests and providing the service.
4. Communicate with the responsible physician—*before* seeing the patient, *during* the evaluation, and *afterward,* with follow-up information.
5. Be practical; give concrete suggestions and avoid theoretical discourses.
6. When things seem confusing, disorganized, overwhelming, or hopeless, organize and lead a case conference for all those involved with the patient.
7. Teach, but do not try to make the requesting physician into a mental health professional.
8. Don't take over primary responsibility for managing the case.
9. Don't expect to work miracles during the crisis of hospitalization; return to baseline functioning is the best outcome that is realistically possible.
10. Always leave a note.

sence of the process in 10 important points that, if followed religiously, will pave the way to Consultants' Heaven.

J. REFERENCES

American Psychiatric Association: Diagnostic and Statistical Manual of Mental Disorders, 3rd Edition, Revised. Washington, DC, American Psychiatric Association, 1987

Balaschak B, Mostofsky D: Seizure disorders, in Behavioral Assessment of Childhood Disorders. Edited by Mash E, Terdal L. New York, Guilford, 1981, pp 601–637

Cohen DJ, Leckman JF, Shaywitz BA: The Tourette syndrome and other tics, in The Clinical Guide to Child Psychiatry. Edited by Shaffer D, Ehrhardt AA, Greenwill L. New York, Free Press, 1984, pp 3–28

Czajkowski DR, Koocher GP: Predicting medical compliance among adolescents with cystic fibrosis. Health Psychol 5:297–305, 1986

Deaton AV: Adaptive noncompliance in pediatric asthma: the parent as expert. J Pediatr Psychol 10:1–14, 1985

Fritz GK, Overholser J: Patterns of response to childhood asthma. Psychosom Med 51:347–355, 1989

Garner DM, Garfinkel PE: The Eating Attitudes Test: an index of the symptoms of anorexia nervosa. Psychol Med 9:273–279, 1979

Garner DM, Olmsted MP, Polivy J: Development and validation of a multidimensional eating disorder inventory for anorexia nervosa and bulimia. International Journal of Eating Disorders 2:15–34, 1983

Harcherick DF, Leckman, JF, Detlor J, et al: A new instrument for clinical studies of Tourette's syndrome. J Am Acad Child Psychiatry 23(2):153–160, 1984

Jackson C, Levine D: Comparison of the Matthews Youth Test for Health and the Hunter-Wolf A-B Rating Scale: measures of Type A behavior in children. Health Psychol 6:255–267, 1987

Kaplan SL, Rosenstein J, Skomorowsky P, et al: The Hospitalized Adolescent Interaction Scale. J Adolesc Health Care 2:101–105, 1981

Koocher G, O'Malley J: The Damocles Syndrome: Psychosocial Consequences of Surviving Childhood Cancer. New York, McGraw-Hill, 1981

Latimer PR: Functional Gastrointestinal Disorders: A Behavioral Medicine Approach. New York, Springer, 1983

McGrath PA: Pain in Children: Nature, Assessment, and Treatment. New York, Guilford, 1990

Rosen JC, Silberg NT, Gross J: Eating Attitudes Test and Eating Disorders Inventory: norms for adolescent girls and boys J Consult Clin Psychol 56:305–308, 1988

Shapiro AK, Shapiro E: Controlled study of pimozide vs. placebo in Tourette's syndrome. J Am Acad Child Psychiatry 23(2):161–173, 1984

Spirito A, Stark LJ, Williams C: Development of a brief coping checklist for use with pediatric populations. J Pediatr Psychol 13:555–574, 1988

Volicer BJ, Bohannon MW: A hospital stress rating scale. Nurs Res 24:352–359, 1975

Walker LS, Greene JW: Children with recurrent abdominal pain and their parents: more somatic complaints, anxiety, and depression than other patient families? J Pediatr 14:231–243, 1989

Wisniewski JJ, Naglieri JA, Mulick JA: Psychometric properties of a Children's Psychosomatic Symptom Checklist. J Behav Med 11:497–507, 1988

Wolf TM, Sklou MC, Wenzl PA, et al: Validation of a measure of type A behavior pattern in children: Bogalusa Heart Study. Child Dev 53:126–135, 1982

Appendix 2–1.   Selected Instruments for Use With Pediatric Patients

Instrument	Brief description	References
Child Somatization Inventory	A 36-item scale that assesses a variety of common somatic complaints; child and parent version availables; some norms are available from the authors.	Walker and Greene 1989
Children's Psychosomatic Symptom Checklist	A 12-item self-report scale for children describing a number of common somatic symptoms (e.g., feeling dizzy, headaches).	Wisniewski et al. 1988
The Hospitalized Adolescent Interaction Scale (HAIS)	A 30-item observer checklist designed to assess the behavior of adolescents in the hospital.	Kaplan et al. 1981
A Hospital Stress Rating Scale	A 49-item checklist devised for adults listing stressful events experienced in the hospital (e.g., being awakened in the night, bad food), many of which are appropriate for children.	Volicer and Bohannon 1975
Kidcope	A 10-item checklist measuring common behavioral and cognitive coping strategies; can be adapted for any treatment or disease-related stressor.	Spirito et al. 1988
The Medical Compliance Incomplete Stories Test	Five incomplete stories read to children involving a decision about whether or not to follow specific medical advice.	Czajkowski and Koocher 1986
Adaptiveness Rating Scale	An 8-item interviewer rating scale designed to assess whether a parent's decision to comply fully with a medical regimen is an adaptive decision.	Deaton 1985
Pain Assessment Measures for Children and Parents	A comprehensive set of parent and child assessment measures designed to assess acute pain (e.g., secondary to medicalprocedures) and chronic pain (e.g., headaches).	(see McGrath 1990)
Children's Asthma Symptom Checklist	Self-report description of symptoms (physical and psychological) experienced during asthma attack.	Fritz and Overholser 1989

Appendix 2–1.   Selected Instruments *(continued)*

Instrument	Brief description	References
Matthews Youth Test for Health (MYTH)	An 18-item parent-teacher rating scale of a child's type A behavior.	(see Jackson and Levine 1987)
Hunter-Wolf A-B Rating Scale	A 24-item self-report scale on type A behavior in children.	Wolf et al. 1982
Digestive Symptoms Inventory	A 52-item interview covering a wide range of bowel symptoms—devised for adults, but most items are suitable for children.	(see Latimer 1983)
Eating Attitudes Test and Eating Disorders Inventory	Two tests commonly used to assess attitudes and behavior characteristics of people with eating disorders. (For adolescent norms, see Rosen et al. 1988.)	Rosen et al. 1988; Garner and Garfinkel 1979; Garner et al. 1983
Tourette Syndrome Severity Scale	A 5-item clinician rating scale.	Shapiro and Shapiro 1984
Tourette Syndrome Global Scale	An observer–clinician-rated scale of tic symptoms and social functioning, each rated on a 100-point scale.	Harcherick et al. 1984
Tourette Syndrome Symptoms List	A 41-item parent-related scale to collect daily ratings of tic behaviors.	Cohen et al. 1984
The Seizure Disorders Survey Schedule (SDSS)	Detailed interview on medical history, characteristics of the seizures, seizure precipitants, and so on.	Balaschak and Mostofsky 1981
Anticipatory Grief Rating Scale	A 4-item interviewer rating scale designed to assess the degree of anticipatory grief in a parent of a child with a life-threatening illness.	Koocher and O'Malley 1981
Appropriateness of Parent-Child Relationship	An 11-item interviewer rating scale designed to assess a variety of behaviors (e.g., protectiveness, discipline) exhibited by parents of a child with a chronic and\or life-threatening illness.	Koocher and O'Malley 1981

CHAPTER THREE

Common Clinical Problems in Pediatric Consultation

Gregory K. Fritz, M.D.

Mental health consultants in a children's hospital encounter a vast range of clinical problems. Psychological factors affect every aspect of the disease process in virtually all pediatric disorders. The clinical domain of consultation-liaison work in pediatrics includes psychophysiologic reactions, psychosomatic disorders, comorbidity, stress responses, noncompliance, adjustment problems, ward management issues, drug interactions, somatization disorders, organic brain syndromes, and ethical dilemmas. A considerable body of literature—both empirical studies and case descriptions—pertains to these clinical problems. Much more work has been done with adults than children, and the results are of varying relevance to the pediatric population. A thorough discussion of each content area that is important to mental health professionals working in pediatrics (as opposed to the process of consultation) is beyond the scope of this book. However, some of the most common clinical problems that confront the consultant in pediatrics are examined in this chapter. Children's responses to hospitalization and living with a chronic illness, pain management, noncompliance, the difficult parent, protocol consultations, and the care of the dying child are discussed as representative clinical problems.

A somewhat altered mind-set regarding psychopathology is required of the child psychiatrist or psychologist working in a children's hospital. Although significant psychopathology certainly does not protect a child from physical illness or the likelihood of pediatric hospitalization (in fact, the reverse may be true), many patients referred for consultation will be found to have relatively mild psychopathology or no diagnosable disorder at all. The consultant who, on coming to such a diagnostic conclusion, infers that there must be no need for a mental health professional's involvement does a disservice to the patient and leaves the pediatric treatment team frustrated. In contrast, the sudden, devastating nature of many pediatric illnesses and the profound disruption of normal life brought about by hospitalization and medical treatment may result in one form or another of decompensation in a previously high-functioning child or family. Such decompensation, although painful and clearly requiring psychosocial intervention, does not have the same prognostic implication as a comparable level of dysfunction in psychiatrically hospitalized children or their families. One encounters a greater range of ego strength in a pediatric hospital than in a psychiatric hospital because a larger proportion of referred pediatric patients are fundamentally sound psychologically.

A. RESPONSE TO HOSPITALIZATION

Every child reacts to the experience of illness and hospitalization, although the nature of the response varies with the child's age and developmental level. Mrazek (1986) discussed in detail the stress responses to pediatric hospitalization exhibited by children at different developmental ages, but a summary is relevant here because of the ubiquitous nature of such responses in hospital consultation work.

1. Infancy

For the infant, hospitalization threatens the developing parent-child attachment. Particular stresses include separation from the parent, the sudden prominence of strangers in the form of medical staff, disruption of the predictable schedule that helped regulate the infant's physiological and psychological activity, and intrusive, painful procedures that tax the infant's sense of trust in the world as a safe and caring environment. Feeding problems, excessive irritability, crying, apathy, withdrawal, or a disturbance in the parent-child relationship are symptoms that may be identified by sensitive staff as indicative of an infant's difficulty in adjusting to hospitalization. Parents faced with the diagnosis of physical disability or illness in their baby typically react with mingled guilt, anger, grief, and denial. The transition to an adaptive, realistic view of their infant's problem is rarely smooth. Preventing chronic dysfunction, such as the "vulnerable child syndrome" (Green and Solnit 1964) can be an important aspect of mental health consultation with very young children.

2. Toddlerhood

Preschoolers' egocentrism and magical thinking make them prone to view illness, hospitalization, and surgery as punishment for real or imagined wrongdoing. Their developmentally appropriate avenues for emotional discharge through motor activity may be restricted by casts, bed rest, or other aspects of hospitalization. Parents' confusion or guilt may lead to inconsistent and ineffective discipline, with resultant behavior problems on the ward prompting a request for consultation.

3. School Age

School-age children have the ability to reason concretely and are more observant of their own body and its functioning. They need and use factual information about their illness, but adults may assume that they are able to conceptualize things more abstractly than is actually the case. Anxiety arising from misunderstanding due to a school-age child's concrete interpretation of medical explanations is common in a pediatric hospital, as the following case example illustrates:

A 9-year-old boy diagnosed as having diabetes mellitus a month previously and already on his third admission was referred for consultation. He was described as anxious, whiny, and uncooperative with every aspect of his treatment. The consultant approached the evaluation in a low-key manner, talking at length with the boy about his collection of baseball trading cards, his desire for a puppy, and other age-appropriate, nonthreatening topics. The child seemed to appreciate the focus on his strengths and interests rather than his illness. Only in their second meeting did the conversation come around to the medical problems. The consultant learned that the boy thought he had "die-a-beets." His understanding was that God had put dead and dying beets in his abdomen, but he could not align his insulin shots and diet restrictions with this explanation of his problem. Basic diabetic education was reinstituted on an individual basis by a nurse with whom he could discuss and clarify his misconceptions. His anxiety decreased significantly, and he became an effective participant in his treatment.

Mastery, learning, and achievement are central tasks for the school-age child. Hospitalization usually interferes with these tasks, resulting, at least transiently, in frustration, resentment, and lowered self-esteem.

4. Adolescence

Adolescents often view illness and hospitalization as an affront to their autonomy. Noncompliance with the medical regimen may result when the illness and its treatment become the battlefield in a teenager's struggle for independence. The pediatric ward and staff are frequently uncomfortable with some aspects of normal adolescent behavior. Especially problematic for a staff used to dealing with prepubertal children is the adolescents' sexuality, which appears—sometimes in exaggerated form—in profanity, desire for privacy, and their provocative behavior with peers. When an illness such as cystic fibrosis is associated with delayed development of secondary sexual characteristics, or when physical disability distorts the body, even medical professionals are prone to treat the teenager as immature and asexual. Failure to acknowledge the emerging sexuality of an adolescent

can inhibit tentative sexual exploration or lead to reactionary acting out. The central importance of peer relationships to an
adolescent's development must be consciously recognized and promoted when chronic illness or hospitalization intrudes. In certain
cases, the consultant's most important intervention can be the facil-
itation of in-hospital relationships with other affected adolescents
or arranging for continuity with friends and schoolmates.

B. PSYCHOLOGICAL FACTORS IN CHRONIC ILLNESS

Although emotional disturbances are by no means universal in
chronically ill children and their families, the preponderance of empirical evidence indicates that chronic pediatric illness constitutes a
substantial risk factor for psychological disorder (Lavigne and Faier-
Routman 1992). Psychological problems associated with chronic illness frequently confront the mental health consultant, and a
framework for conceptualizing them is required. We have previously suggested that influential psychological factors be considered at the following phases of the illness process: 1) vulnerability to
disease, 2) symptom onset, 3) recurrence, 4) maintenance of the disease state, and 5) living with or reacting to the illness (Fritz and
Brown 1991). In evaluating an individual patient, the consultant
must remember that a psychosomatic component is at least theoretically possible in every phase of all chronic disorders. It is also possible that, for a given child, the psychological factors are of minimal
importance—even with diseases such as asthma and ulcerative colitis, in which psychosocial components have been widely recognized.
Thorough, open-minded evaluation of the individual child avoids
the clinical errors associated with a cookbook approach.

Vulnerability to disease is increased by behaviors such as smoking,
overeating, and drug abuse. In teenagers, unintentional injuries, homicide, and suicide are the three leading causes of death. A consultant
may help in the identification of vulnerable patients and contribute
preventative efforts in such cases. The precipitation of a *symptom onset*

by psychological factors was probably overemphasized in the past because of the impact of psychosomatic specificity theory. According to this theory, the "holy seven" psychosomatic illnesses—asthma, peptic ulcer, rheumatoid arthritis, ulcerative colitis, neurodermatitis, thyrotoxicosis, and essential hypertension—were thought to be caused by specific emotional conflicts (Alexander 1950). Attachment dysfunction leading to failure to thrive in infancy is perhaps the clearest example of psychosocial stress associated with symptom onset. *Recurrence* or flares in symptomatology in response to psychological stress can be identified as a pattern in subgroups of patients with a variety of chronic illnesses. In patients with diabetes, for example, stressful experiences have been associated with poor short-term and long-term glucose control. Psychological stress or family conflict can precipitate acute asthmatic episodes, and case reports have described frequent emotional triggers of asthma in patients who subsequently died (Fritz et al. 1987).

Psychological factors can contribute to the *maintenance of a disease state* through various mechanisms. The biologic aspects of specific psychological disorders, such as depression or anxiety, may be synergistic with the pathophysiology of a chronic illness such as asthma or hypertension. Diagnosis and proper treatment of the psychiatric disorder will result in concomitant improvement in the patient's chronic disease. Alternatively, intrapsychic factors or family dysfunction may lead to noncompliance and, subsequently, increased morbidity. Even with the same level of physical limitation, two patients with the same illness may demonstrate remarkably different degrees of success in *living with the illness*. Exaggeration of the sick role, poor self-image, symptom preoccupation or magnification, and withdrawal from parts of life that are realistically accessible are unfortunate adjustment outcomes for a chronically ill child. It may be a difficult task for the consultant to determine whether a particular patient's adjustment represents impaired coping or a creative solution to a trying situation. Mattsson (1972) has suggested criteria for what constitutes reasonable adjustment to a pediatric chronic illness:

1. Age-appropriate dependence on the family
2. Minimal need for secondary gain from the illness

3. Acceptance of the limits and responsibilities imposed by the illness
4. The development of compensatory sources of satisfaction

Depression, anxiety, alienation, significant regression, or major conflict should not be written off as inevitable components of a chronic illness. Clinical judgment ultimately defines the need for intervention, and treatable conditions should not be ignored because they occur in the context of chronic physical illness.

C. PAIN

Psychiatrists and psychologists in a pediatric hospital are frequently asked to consult on the management of children's pain. The problem is often presented as "pain in excess of what is organically based" or "rule out functional etiology for the pain." A degree of suspicion or annoyance with the patient often accompanies the staff's referral. Especially with infants and toddlers, physicians have historically underestimated children's capacity to feel pain because of the presumed immaturity of the nervous system. Although there has been considerable progress in recent years, a pain referral usually requires the consultant to deal with an artificial mind-body dualism, inadequate and unsystematic prescription of analgesics, and reliance on purely pharmacologic pain management. A thorough discussion of the treatment of pain is available in several detailed reviews (Masek et al. 1984; Newburger and Sallan 1981); the following overview summarizes issues of particular importance to the consultant.

1. Evaluation of Pain

The assessment of pain in a child is difficult. Even the definition of pain is widely debated. Pain has traditionally been seen as the nervous system's warning signal of tissue damage; greater pain was associated with more extensive damage. This view is now recognized as far too simplistic, because it ignores the psychological components of pain, does not account for the tremendous individual and circumstantial variation in the pain experience, and poorly explains the chronic pain syndrome. Unlike the philosophical debate about whether sound is produced when a tree falls in the woods but there is no one to hear it, pain clearly exists only as a subjective phenomenon. It entails sensation, conscious perception, the expression of suffering, and pain-related behavior changes.

Several approaches have been proposed to help children quantify their pain. In an exhaustive study of pain perception in 994 children of different ages, Ross and Ross (1984) found that most children had difficulty discriminating pain verbally using adjectives they had been given. A visual analog scale anchored in familiar areas of children's experience (e.g., loudness of school sounds) improves assessment validity. Observers' quantification of "distress" behavior is possible through the use of behavior checklists (Katz et al. 1984).

One flawed assessment technique commonly used to differentiate "functional" from "organic" pain is the placebo response. Placebo response involves measurable changes in circulating endorphins, and it occurs in subgroups of every population, including those with overtly demonstrable tissue damage. It is no more common among psychologically disturbed individuals than among those without depression, somatization, hysteria, or another psychiatric diagnosis. The technique of substituting saline for a single analgesic dose and observing a response is a demonstration of conditioning rather than the power of placebo. In short, the placebo response proves only that the patient responds to placebo under particular circumstances—nothing more. Because of the potential damage to the doctor-patient relationship and the lack of definitive information provided, the consultant should discourage the diagnostic use of placebo.

2. Comorbidity

Several psychiatric disorders may be interwoven with pain in a complex cause-and-effect relationship. Depression is frequently associated with pain, often in a reactive way that lowers pain tolerance, magnifies suffering, and aggravates maladaptive pain behavior. Anxiety disorders, when present, may augment the experience of pain; adequate treatment of the anxiety allows more effective coping with the pain that remains. Somatoform disorders are poorly characterized for children at present, but pain—in the form of headache, recurrent abdominal pain, or diffuse pain complaints—is certainly a prominent symptom in patients considered to have one of these diagnoses. Delusional pain as part of a schizophrenic process and the factitious pain of malingering are uncommon but possible presentations in childhood.

3. Principles of Treatment

The consultant dealing with a pain management problem should adhere to several basic principles. Accepting the reality of the suffering and communicating this acceptance in an empathetic manner are essential to all that follows. Medication should be prescribed at regular intervals (not on an as-needed basis) and at doses sufficient to keep the patient pain free. Addiction is rarely a significant problem in pediatric pain patients, in contrast to the frequency with which it influences staff decision making. Analgesics should be prescribed logically, starting with nonnarcotic agents and progressing to narcotics of increasing potency and narcotic adjuvants (antidepressants, neuroleptics, benzodiazepines, anticonvulsants, and antihistamines). Antidepressants have been demonstrated to be useful by themselves in pain management whether or not there are prominent depressive symptoms. The mechanism is not defined, and no particular antidepressant has been found to be more effective than the others. Behavioral approaches are useful in reducing reinforcement of pain and illness behaviors.

Psychophysiological techniques such as biofeedback-enhanced relaxation training can reduce arousal and tension. Increasing a child's communication skills allows him or her to interact more effectively with parents and caretaking staff.

D. NONCOMPLIANCE

The failure of children and their families to adhere to a prescribed pediatric treatment regimen is a serious problem that often elicits a referral for mental health consultation. There is empirical evidence documenting noncompliance rates as high as 90% (Lemanek 1990). Acute illnesses (e.g., otitis media), chronic illnesses (e.g., asthma, diabetes, and arthritis), life-threatening conditions (e.g., renal transplantation and cancer treatment) and surgical problems (e.g., scoliosis rehabilitation) are all adversely affected by treatment noncompliance. A growing body of clinical research seeks to delineate the variables that contribute to noncompliance and to find effective interventions (LaGreca 1990).

Confronted by a request to evaluate a patient whom the medical team reports to be poorly compliant with treatment, the consultant needs to clarify several basic issues. First, what are the details of the regimen that have actually been prescribed to the patient? Have the details of the child's specific treatment been spelled out to the patient and family with regard to what is expected, or has the noncompliance been determined in relation to some implicit, ideal standard of good treatment? Have the patient and family been provided with a single, clear message, or are there conflicting attitudes and instructions that confuse the picture?

Second, the consultant needs to be aware of how the noncompliance is measured. Is it inferred from the fact that the management of the disease process has been difficult? Physiologic changes during the adolescent growth spurt can alter previously stable diabetes, cardiac disease, and seizure disorders despite excellent adherence to the treatment regimen. Is it determined on the basis of parent report? Parents and children have been shown to differ in their descriptions of compliance; children's reports sometimes correlate more closely than parents' with objective measures.

The third issue to be clarified at the outset of the evaluation is the nature of the relationship between the physicians and the patient and family. Is there familiarity, trust, and respect between physician and patient, or is the relationship characterized by suspicion or animosity?

A poor relationship increases the likelihood of noncompliance and reduces the quality of the information used to judge the significance of the noncompliance.

Ideally, the consultant's suggested intervention is based on the factors found to be underlying the noncompliance for a particular child and family. Inadequate knowledge is frequently associated with noncompliance. In complicated treatment protocols, such as those associated with severe asthma or brittle diabetes, good knowledge about one aspect of the illness does not necessarily predict adequate knowledge about other aspects. Theoretical knowledge does not ensure sufficient skill in using an inhaler or testing urine (in which high rates of error are the rule). Children's understanding of the illness and its treatment must be reevaluated and repeated as their social and intellectual capacities mature. Noncompliance may be a manifestation of individual or family psychopathology, as the following case example illustrates:

> Luis was a 15-year-old Mexican-American boy whose remission of acute lymphocytic leukemia was threatened by noncompliance with his oral methotrexate regimen. Although he was pleasant and cooperative in other respects, his blood levels of methotrexate were nondetectable. In an extended evaluation with the psychiatric consultant, Luis described extreme dysfunction in his family: his father and brothers got drunk and fought, his young sister was pregnant, and his mother was seriously depressed. Direct questioning revealed that his noncompliance was suicidal, as his intent was to die of leukemia. In his words, "If I die, maybe they will get serious and straighten up. If they go down, well, I'll go down with them. . . . " Luis began formal psychiatric treatment, and community resources were mobilized in a partially successful effort to help his family. Luis successfully completed his treatment before being lost to follow-up.

Finally, noncompliance may be a symptom of excessive denial in a patient who cannot come to terms with the seriousness of the illness. It may also stem from inadequate social skills to deal with awkward times among peers, lack of an organized family structure to provide needed supervision, or insufficient motivation in the patient, the family, or both. More detailed intervention approaches are described in the following chapter.

E. THE DIFFICULT PARENT

Hospitalized children usually have one or more parental figures involved in their care. Most often, these adults are the central supports for the child, "interpreting" in both directions for the medical team and the child, eliciting the child's cooperation, and facilitating the treatment in multiple ways. At times, however, the parents may impede treatment or alienate the staff to a degree that a mental health consultation is requested for "parent management." The child psychiatrist or psychologist should resist the temptation to pass the request on to the adult consult service ("because the real patient is an adult") and recognize that helping the pediatric staff interact successfully with a child's parents is a task of critical importance.

The specific consultation request often conveys little beyond the staff's frustration and annoyance with the parent. The job of the consultant is to provide a more subtle description of the specific characterological or psychopathologic features that underlie the difficult or obnoxious behavior and then suggest a management strategy. Several important articles (Groves 1975; Kahana and Bibring 1965) deal with personality factors as they affect the medical management of adult patients in the general hospital. The ideas presented are readily applied to work with parents whose children are hospitalized, and these articles can be as useful to the pediatric team as they are to the mental health consultant. Although it is important to recognize and differentiate specific personality patterns, the consultant should avoid any attempt to alter or treat the characterological problems of parents whose children are hospitalized. The high level of stress related to the child's illness, the lack of any desire for psychological treatment on the parents' part, and the staff's lack of psychological expertise together ensure that efforts to bring about character change on a pediatric ward are doomed. Parental character styles are identified to enable staff to "go *with* the grain rather than *against* it" in interactions with the parent.

Parents with a predominantly dependent character structure present the pediatric staff with a barrage of needy requests that frequently turn into demands when they are not satisfied. The staff become exhausted and then angry; withdrawal and avoidance only intensify the demand for attention. After describing the pattern and clarifying and validating the staff's feelings, the consultant most importantly aids the staff in setting limits that still convey caring. Structured contact times, frequent but brief interactions, and concerned reassurance are especially helpful.

Parents with a more compulsive style are prone to end up in control struggles with staff and to be seen as rigid, intellectualized, and unemotional. Discussion of the importance of compulsive defenses to manage overwhelming anxiety often helps the staff approach these parents with more empathy even if the parents' affect remains isolated. Scientific explanations, background reading, and involvement (to a degree) in decision making are emphasized in staff interactions with compulsive parents. Monitoring intake and output, counting calories, and so forth help the parents feel that they have some control over the treatment their child is receiving.

The parent with a borderline personality disorder presents a major challenge to the pediatric unit because of intense affect, impulsiveness, and a tendency to split staff into all-good and all-bad categories. Ineffective interactions with the parent, compromised patient care, and significant conflict among the professionals often have progressed quite far by the time the consultant enters such a case. The detailed description by Groves (1978) of the general hospital management of the borderline character is as relevant today as it was a decade ago. The consultant helps the staff to avoid the good/bad split through clear, consistent communication, to deal with the parent's pervasive sense of entitlement while avoiding confrontation with it, and to set firm limits that are consistent with normal ward functioning.

Parents with significant psychopathology, such as depression, schizophrenia, or alcoholism, need to be involved in appropriate treatment. The consultant acts as a "go-between" in these cases, arranging referrals and providing feedback to the staff. The consultant also supports a calm, businesslike, common-sense approach toward this parent on the part of the staff.

F. PROTOCOL CONSULTATIONS

A mark of an established consultation-liaison service is the existence of protocols whereby all patients with a specific disorder automatically receive a mental health consultation. Patient groups for whom such protocol referrals are often instituted include hospitalized persons who have attempted suicide, newly diagnosed patients with serious chronic illnesses such as cancer or diabetes, failure-to-thrive infants, and transplantation candidates. There are many advantages to having such protocols in place:

1. Mental health involvement is made routine and universal, thus eliminating the perception that the patient will be stigmatized by having contact with a psychiatrist or psychologist.
2. Contact is made early, allowing prevention of significant dysfunction through education, ventilation, and timely intervention.
3. No patient "falls through the cracks" through oversight or missed communication.
4. Psychosocial issues assume a higher priority for the medical team when there is regular input from mental health professionals.
5. Financial reimbursement for consultation occurs more reliably.
6. Clinical research on the target population is facilitated with a good baseline assessment.

Establishment of consultation protocols depends on two critical elements: 1) a solid, mutually respectful relationship between the pediatric team and the consultation-liaison service and 2) a cadre of experienced, interested mental health professionals available to carry out the evaluations on a timely basis. The consultant conducting an assessment of a child and family referred by protocol usually has a standard outline of the procedure to follow. The challenge is to carry out the assessment in a standard fashion without letting it become rote or clinically mindless.

Patients who have attempted suicide are the group for whom a consultation is most frequently required as part of the pediatric hospitalization, probably because the need is so obvious when self-injury is severe enough to merit medical hospitalization. The primary task is to determine the level of lethality, both immediately and after stabilization. To do so, the consultant must confront the nature of the attempt with the patient and elicit the thoughts, feelings, and actions surrounding it, as well as assess the family and environmental resources. The desire to establish a positive alliance or to begin psychotherapy takes a back seat to the need for a focused evaluation. Self-report instruments, such as the Children's Depression Inventory, the Suicide Intent Scale, or the Hopelessness Scale for Children, augment the clinical interview and may provide additional data. The consultant should promptly assume responsibility for determining the level of care needed, especially whether constant observation is indicated. The acute pediatric ward, with its bustling activity, lack of privacy, and medical orientation, is a surprisingly safe place for most patients who have attempted suicide. In-hospital repeat suicide attempts are vanishingly rare on pediatric units with effective consultation-liaison services.

G. THE DYING CHILD

The death of a child is widely recognized as one of the most difficult aspects of medical care for pediatric staff. The dying child has been deprived of most of life's experiences and thus has a small store of memories and accomplishments to reflect on. Children have fewer cognitive resources to use in coping with the reality of death, and the inevitable loneliness of dying is especially difficult for a child who is so dependent on adult caretakers. Death before fulfillment may be particularly hard for many physicians to tolerate because of the delayed gratification they have imposed on themselves in their own professional training. Many pediatricians selected pediatrics at least partly because they sought to avoid caring for dying patients. Those who entered medicine to master death find that their omnipotence is reinforced by medical training. The action orientation of most pediatricians and the ready availability of high-technology medicine at times seem to conspire to remove the pediatric staff from close involvement with the dying child. Despite the fact that their own patients' illnesses are rarely fatal, psychiatrists and psychologists are frequently consulted when a patient is dying because the staff hope that they will have something unique to offer to the terminally ill child and the family.

In the past, adults have tended to believe that, because children do not verbalize a great deal about death, they are not concerned or knowledgeable about it. Certainly, it is hard to know how death affects a preverbal infant or toddler, but the commonly observed peek-a-boo games and fascination with dead insects may reflect concern about being versus nonbeing. Preoperational children approximately 3–6 years of age see death as a different but reversible circumstance in life during which there may still be some functioning. Thus, at a pet's funeral the author's 4-year-old wanted to bury some lettuce for his dead turtle to eat. School-age children with concrete operational thought processes recognize that death is final and irreversible, but view it as external and not necessarily inevitable. As children move into adolescence, their concepts of death approach those of adults.

Life experiences interact with the child's cognitive level of development to produce an understanding of death that is unique to the particular child. Seriously ill children have had closer contact with death, which is often reflected in an understanding that is different from and more mature than that of healthy children. Their view of illness, prognosis, and death evolves gradually, affected by the information they are given (both overtly and covertly), by exposure to the deaths of other patients, and by the course of their illnesses. Some terminally ill children can't discuss their feelings about death. They may, however, reveal their awareness in comments such as "I won't be going back to school" or "I'll miss my sister's birthday." Some unusual behaviors make sense when they are understood in the context of death awareness, such as waning interest in future nice things, distancing of important individuals, or a fear of wasting time. Many terminally ill children perceive unspoken rules—such as "avoid painful topics" or "let people pretend things are not so bad"—and act on them even at considerable psychological expense, as the following case example illustrates:

Linda was a 13-year-old girl with non-Hodgkin's lymphoma for whom all treatment options had been exhausted. Her wasted body, frequent bleeding, mouth sores, and bone pain made every day more miserable. Because of her fundamentalist religious beliefs, Linda's mother was convinced that a miracle would happen if their hearts were pure and they prayed enough. She'd organized her church to hold prayer services and urged her daughter to focus on praying for a miracle. Linda dutifully complied, but the nurses were concerned that her own needs were not being met, and a consultation was requested.

In individual discussions with the consultant, Linda readily revealed an accurate awareness of her situation and a desire to give up the struggle. She felt she shouldn't reveal these feelings to her mother or assert her wishes because "my mother can't stand the thought of losing me." She worried that she wouldn't have the energy to keep up the pretense, and she tearfully wished that she could again be close to her mother.

The consultant continued to meet with Linda regularly until she died 2 weeks later. Her grief, fears, memories, and final desires were the substance of these meetings, and the consultant promised that she would try to help her mother after Linda died. Efforts to restore the intimacy of the mother-daughter relationship in its final days were partially successful.

The consultant may have a great deal to contribute to the management of some dying children and little to contribute in other cases, even on the same unit with consistent staff. Guilt lurks everywhere when a child faces death—in the staff for their failure to cure, in the parents for not protecting their child or for looking forward to the release of death, and in the child for making others feel bad. The consultant may need to help people confront, examine, and move beyond their irrational guilt. Withdrawal from the dying child takes many forms—avoiding the room on rounds, superficial interactions, preoccupation with technical details—but it always makes the child frightened and isolated. The pediatric team and the parents may be in a dilemma about how far to press treatment, and the consultant may serve to facilitate an effective conference or to elicit the patient's wishes to help resolve the issue. Recognition of the dying child's psychological needs may result in the consultant helping the child to write or tape-record important feelings or messages, arranging for meaningful goodbyes, or reassuring the child that beloved people or pets will be cared for. Consultation work with terminally ill patients is emotionally draining, but the effort makes it possible for the child, the family, and the staff to deal with the death in a dignified and compassionate manner.

H. CONCLUSION

This chapter summarizes available information on some of the clinical problems common to consultation-liaison work in pediatrics. The topics covered represent only a portion of the clinical spectrum encountered; indeed, the wide range of the presenting problems and the complexity of the medical system together produce an extraordinary variety of clinical challenges. Every medical advance—whether it is transplantation, total parenteral nutrition, self-management of chronic illness, reconstructive plastic surgery, or progress in the neonatal intensive care unit—has associated psychological stresses for the patient and the family. Specific illnesses, such as hemophilia, asthma, muscular dystrophy, and regional enteritis, have unique psychosomatic components and at the same time have many characteristics in common with pediatric chronic illness. The pediatric consultation-liaison arena presents numerous opportunities for creative clinical research to advance our knowledge of how psychological factors affect children's diseases and their treatment. The effective consultant must be familiar with current clinical and empirical research on a particular problem and also must apply experience from other psychological realms to the pediatric setting. It is this combination that spells clinical wisdom.

I. REFERENCES

Alexander F: Psychosomatic Medicine: Its Principles and Application. New York, WW Norton, 1950

Fritz GK, Brown LK: Concept and Classification of Psychosomatic Disorders, in Textbook of Child and Adolescent Psychiatry. Edited by Wiener JM. Washington, DC, American Psychiatric Press, 1991, pp 422–430

Fritz GK, Rubenstein S, Lewiston NJ: Psychological factors in fatal childhood asthma. Am J Orthopsychiatry 57:253–257, 1987

Green M, Solnit AJ: Reactions to the threatened loss of a child: a vulnerable child syndrome. Pediatrics 34:58–66, 1964

Groves JE: Management of the borderline patient on a medical or surgical ward: the psychiatric consultant's role. Int J Psychiatry Med 6:337–348, 1975

Groves JE: Taking care of the hateful patient. N Engl J Med 298:883–887, 1978

Kahana RJ, Bibring GL: Personality types and medical management, in Psychiatry and Medical Practice in a General Hospital. Edited by Zinberg NE. Madison, CT, International Universities Press, 1965, pp 108–123

Katz ER, Varni JW, Jay SM: Behavioral assessment and management of pediatric pain. Prog Behav Modif 18:163–193, 1984

LaGreca AM: Issues in adherence with pediatric regimens. J Pediatr Psychol 15:423–436, 1990

Lavigne JV, Faier-Routman J: Psychological adjustment to pediatric physical disorders: a meta-analytic review. J Pediatr Psychology 17:133–157, 1992

Lemanek K: Adherence issues in the medical management of asthma. J Pediatr Psychol 15:437–458, 1990

Masek BJ, Russo DC, Varni JW: Behavioral approaches to the management of chronic pain in children. Pediatr Clin North Am 31:1113–1132, 1984

Mattsson A: Long-term physical illness in childhood: a challenge to psychosocial adaptation. Pediatrics 52:801–811, 1972

Mrazek D: Pediatric hospitalization: understanding the stress from a developmental perspective, in The Psychosomatic Approach: Contemporary Practice of Whole-Person Care. Edited by Christie M, Mellett P. New York, Wiley, 1986, pp 164–196

Newburger PE, Sallan SE: Chronic pain: principles of management. J Pediatr 98:180–189, 1981

Ross DM, Ross SA: The importance of type of question, psychological climate and subject set in interviewing children about pain. Pain 19:71–79, 1984

CHAPTER FOUR

Psychological Interventions for Pediatric Patients

Anthony Spirito, Ph.D.
Gregory K. Fritz, M.D.

The mental health consultant to a pediatric unit provides a psychological evaluation of the child and the family that leads to a diagnosis and formulation of the significant psychosocial factors in the case. Sometimes all that the pediatric treatment team needs or desires is for the consultant to make a diagnosis. More often, however, the evaluation points to the need for an intervention that the consultant must recommend, arrange, or provide. Failure to follow through with ongoing involvement, to "get one's hands dirty," will result in the consultant being viewed as ineffectual, elitist, or disinterested. The consultant should be aware of the full range of interventions that are useful for the psychological problems of pediatric patients.

In addition to improving patient care, consultants who can be therapeutically useful will derive more professional satisfaction from consultation-liaison work than those who are limited to diagnostic "hit-and-run" missions. In this chapter, we discuss a spectrum of interventions, from educational approaches to psychiatric hospitalization, that may be required by the child, the parents or family, or the pediatric staff.

A. EDUCATION OF PATIENTS AND PARENTS

Education plays a particularly important role in managing acutely hospitalized children and children with a newly diagnosed disease. It is important to assess how much the patient and family know and understand about the illness. Fantasies about the etiology, prognosis, and expected course of an illness are common among pediatric patients (including adolescents) and their parents. Such fantasies combined with a fertile imagination may be more psychologically disabling than the disorder itself. Education about the illness and its implications helps the patient by replacing fantasy with fact and supporting intellectual defenses as a means of coping. Parents also need to be educated about typical responses of children to different invasive treatment procedures, possible psychological effects of hospitalization or chronic illness at different developmental stages, behavioral effects of certain medications, and other common emotional sequelae.

1. Invasive Medical Procedures

Educating parents about the way in which children respond to invasive medical procedures can help allay the parents' own anxieties and alleviate their guilt about the child's difficulty in adapting to these procedures. It is helpful to assess the child's previous response to stressful medical procedures and place the child's behavior in that context. The most practical distinction for parents is that between two general coping styles: 1) children who *actively engage* in various behaviors to manage the stress associated with the medical procedure and 2) children who tend to *avoid* the negative aspects of the procedure. It is useful to explain to parents how some children do better by watching procedures, whereas other children do better by closing their eyes. Advice to parents about how children best tolerate procedures (e.g., by using simple breathing techniques and other types of active coping) may enhance their skills as "coaches."

2. Psychological Effects of Illness or Hospitalization

Explaining the psychological impact of illness or hospitalization at different ages (see Chapter 2) is often useful; several articles (e.g., Magrab 1985; Willis et al. 1982) contain descriptions of reactions at different ages. Specific examples of a child's behavior that reflect an underlying developmental theme can be clarified for parents. For example, when the reaction of an adolescent to illness is discussed, it is important for the parents to understand the effects of illness on the adolescent's striving for independence. Parents often attempt to soothe an adolescent who is hospitalized or assume caretaker responsibility. Adolescents predictably respond negatively to such actions, which they see as overprotective. In such cases, resentment may develop between parent and adolescent.

3. Behavioral Effects of Medications

Parents should be aware of the behavioral effects of certain medications. One of the medications that most commonly concerns parents is prednisone; several articles (Drigan et al. 1992; Harris et al. 1986; Ling et al. 1981) describe the behavioral effects of steroids at different dosages. Even if the pediatrician has described the behavioral effects of steroids, it is useful for the consultant to review them. Parents may have concerns and (unfounded) fears about permanent behavioral changes after discontinuation of the prednisone.

When children are treated with narcotics, parents often have concerns about addiction. Parents may get mixed signals from the pediatric team that manages their child's pain. Some physicians are reluctant to increase the dosage of narcotics because they fear addiction and may convey their reluctance to the parents. Even when physicians are not concerned about addiction, parents may be. It is helpful to explain to parents that addiction is very rare (Schecter 1985) and that a child's pain may be undertreated because of fear of addiction.

4. Beliefs About Illness and the Medical Regimen

Assessment of the patient's and the family's beliefs about the illness or the treatment regimen, or both, may reveal important misconceptions. If, for example, the patient has unexpressed doubts about the effectiveness of the medication regimen being prescribed for asthma, then the patient is at significant risk for noncompliance. A consultant's assessment can help the health care staff to convey information effectively and can enhance compliance, as illustrated in the following case example:

> Consultation was requested by the mother of a 2-year-old boy with asthma because she could not get him to swallow his oral medications. She described fruitless games, bribes, and battles; her lack of success was reflected in low blood levels of the medication and poor asthma control. The consultant arrived at the child's bed at the same time as the father, who was reported to be unhelpful and uninvolved with the child's care. Able to interview both parents for the history of the problem, the consultant quickly elicited from the father (who was audibly wheezing himself) his belief that his son did not have asthma and did not need medication any more than he did. Moreover, he felt his wife and the female pediatrician were going to make the child view himself as sickly with their emphasis on asthma and medicine. He refused to help his wife in the management of a disease whose existence he denied in his son (as well as himself), although he was caring and involved with his son in other ways. The pediatrician and the consultant worked together to help the father confront his fears and his misinformation as the critical step in improving the child's asthma treatment.

5. Educational Programs

A number of advocacy groups sponsor educational programs related to the illness that is their concern. Local chapters of the American Lung Association, the Cystic Fibrosis Foundation, the Ileitis and Colitis Foundation, the Celiac Society, the Hemophilia Foundation, and others disseminate information through meetings, speakers, discussion groups, newsletters, and other written materials. They are a valuable and underused resource. We have reviewed the characteristics of educational programs that successfully promote self-management of asthma and concluded that the extensive experience with asthma can be generalized to other illnesses (Fritz 1987).

Successful programs make the children and their parents sophisticated partners with the physician in managing the illness and enhancing normal functioning. Information is presented about the etiology, course, prognosis, and treatment of the disease. Both professionals and experienced patients are available to field questions. Good educational programs consider the developmental level of the children, as well as the parents' needs.

B. EDUCATION OF STAFF

In liaison work, the mental health consultant focuses on the pediatric staff rather than on a particular patient or family. Through an ongoing, collaborative relationship, the consultant seeks to increase the psychosocial knowledge, sensitivity, and clinical skills of the professionals. *Liaison* activities have been compared to direct *consultation* in an ongoing debate in the literature about the appropriate role of mental health professionals in the pediatric hospital. In practice, one is rarely confronted with the need to make an either/or decision between consultation and liaison interventions (Fritz 1990). Liaison primarily involves education and takes various forms. Education of health care staff can play an important role in improving the staff-patient relationship. Teaching the nursing and medical staff about the psychological effects of hospitalization, adaptation to chronic illness, and patients' beliefs about illness is a useful consultative function. Such teaching often occurs around a particular case as the consultant explains the origin of certain behaviors or beliefs. Nursing and medical staff put the patient's behavior into better perspective, which, in turn, affects the care the patient receives.

When more formal teaching is needed, the consultant may initiate or lead a time-limited in-service program on a topic of interest to medical or nursing staff. When a consultant has a liaison relationship with a pediatric subspecialty team, education can also occur at a regular weekly or monthly meeting in which psychosocial issues are discussed. Such meetings often help to alleviate the stress experienced in the care of a particular patient.

A number of excellent clinical articles describe the psychological facets of specific diseases or the problems commonly encountered in medical settings. Such readings can be helpful to nursing and medical staff. Experienced consultants have a collection of such articles and papers that reflect their own approach to patient management.

The medical team may require considerable support from the consultant in a liaison capacity, especially when patient or family behavior is difficult to manage and the nursing and medical staff become upset with the patient. In such circumstances, the consultant may serve as a mediator between medical personnel and patients to ensure an adequate working relationship. Control battles often arise between health care professionals and adolescents regarding the medical regimen or hospital stay. The consultant can help the health care staff anticipate conflicts and thus help normalize some of the adolescents' reactions. When stresses arise, case conferences and individual meetings with health care professionals can reframe patient behaviors as psychologically meaningful and thereby lessen angry feelings of the health care staff toward the patient, as illustrated in the following case example:

> Ms. A, the mother of an 8-year-old girl newly diagnosed as having leukemia, quickly became involved in fund-raising activities for the local Leukemia Society. When her daughter was hospitalized, she frequently tried to recruit parents whose children also had cancer to become fund-raisers for the Society. Ms. A made her appeals in a loud and demanding manner, which was successful in raising money outside the hospital, but often had a negative effect on the other parents. Many of these parents, who were spending long hours in the hospital with their children, felt guilty about not participating in fund-raising. The nursing staff became angry at Ms. A for being "insensitive" and upsetting the other parents; they suggested that she be severely restricted from talking with other parents on the floor and not be allowed on the unit if she did not adhere to the restriction.

A meeting was held between nursing staff and the consultant after an evaluation was completed. The consultant reframed Ms. A's fund-raising activities as a means for her to cope with feelings of helplessness in the face of her daughter's illness. Her insensitivity was construed as a measure of her desperation. In discussing the case, the nurses were able to modify their punitive attitude. A plan was devised wherein the consultant discussed with Ms. A the impact of her behavior on other parents and began the limit-setting processes. Individual nurses discussed with the other parents ways that they might assert themselves if they felt uncomfortable in their interactions with Ms. A. Together, their interventions led to a decrease in the stressful interactions between Ms. A and the other parents on the floor.

Conflicts between health care professionals and pediatric patients more often arise when the patients are chronically ill rather than acutely ill. Caring for chronically ill children can be stressful for staff, and the stress can affect the patients either directly or indirectly. For example, if health care professionals have worked closely with a child who is dying, the threat of loss may be so intense that they withdraw from the patient during the end stage of disease. Such withdrawal can have negative effects on the parents and the patient. Other issues for medical teams who care for chronically ill children have been reviewed by Bronheim and Jacobstein (1984).

C. INTERVENTION WITH PARENTS

Formal psychological intervention is often necessary to affect the behavior of parents or staff. Education is a necessary first step and sets the stage for subsequent interventions. A number of interventions can be provided for the adults in a pediatric setting and should regularly be considered by the consultant.

1. Supportive Psychotherapy for Parents

Brief, supportive interventions for parents are common and cost-effective in a pediatric hospital. A well-functioning parent is the single most important psychological resource for a sick child. Supportive psychotherapy may be helpful to parents who are having difficulty adjusting to a child's illness. Helping a parent cope with psychologically threatening information about a child's illness can play an important role in the overall management of the patient. Supportive psychotherapy usually focuses on the distress that accompanies hospitalization or a serious diagnosis. Encouraging parents to become actively involved in the child's care and in medical decisions regarding their child is another goal of supportive psychotherapy. Support groups for parents can be helpful in addition to, or instead of, individual interventions. The consultant should be aware of the organizations and their contact persons in the community who provide such support.

Supportive psychotherapy is perceived by some mental health professionals as below the level of training they have obtained to treat difficult psychological problems. Clinicians need to bear in mind that supportive psychotherapy requires listening and empathic skills, the cornerstones of all psychotherapeutic work. The consultant often deals with psychologically healthy parents who find themselves in extremely stressful situations. Relatively brief supportive sessions can make a major difference. The consultant may also arrange for supportive psychotherapy to be provided by other hospital staff such as social workers or clergy.

2. Family Therapy

Family therapy may be recommended by the consultant as the treatment of choice to help a child and his or her parents adapt to a threatening diagnosis or a difficult, prolonged hospitalization. Family therapy includes the siblings and appraises the reactions of all family members. Significant problems are identified and managed early. The consultant can alert the family to the effect of the diagnosis on other family members, particularly the siblings. The consultant can assist the family's coping efforts by bringing up concerns about the siblings to try to prevent them from occurring; for example, the consultant could explain that siblings may exhibit stress through somatic complaints or dysfunction in school (Lobato 1990). A consultant should also evaluate the social network, sociocultural influences, and adaptive style of the family of a newly diagnosed patient, as in the following case example:

> A consultant was called to the pediatric intensive care unit to evaluate suicidality in a mother of a terminally ill patient. The mother was Cambodian and had emigrated several years earlier. An interpreter was needed to conduct the evaluation, which revealed a horrific personal history of trauma and death. This mother experienced the death of a young child from disease and the murder of her entire family during the Khmer Rouge takeover of Cambodia. The mother had been away from the village when the slaughter by the Khmer Rouge occurred. On seeing her murdered family, she apparently went into a state of shock and wandered for months through the countryside. She eventually ended up in a refugee camp in Thailand and emigrated to the United States from the camp. Once in this country, she married another Cambodian refugee and started another family. Her second child from this second family was subsequently diagnosed with leukemia and was now terminally ill. She strongly believed that the impending loss of this child, in the context of the deaths of her other children, meant that she must be unfit as a parent and was a sign that she herself should be dead. When her child died, she said that she would leave the hospital immediately and wander the streets until she died, a recreation of her previous experience in Cambodia.
>
> After speaking with the Southeast Asian relief organization to familiarize himself with aspects of Cambodian culture, the consultant met with the family patriarch and members of the extended family. The family members agreed to be in close contact with this woman and her family after the death of the child to ensure that she didn't leave her family. This plan helped to avert an immediate crisis. At 3-month follow-up, the mother was still actively grieving but was not suicidal and remained at home attending to the needs of her remaining child to the best of her ability.

Significant family conflicts and family dysfunction can impede a child's care, and family therapy may be necessary for the smooth medical management of the child. When the family's pre-existing psychological difficulties are compounded by the stress associated with the illness, therapy can be both difficult and time-consuming. Strong family therapy skills are necessary to manage such patients and families. Consultants for whom family therapy is not a comfortable treatment modality should develop competent referral resources.

D. INDIVIDUAL INTERVENTIONS FOR PEDIATRIC PATIENTS

1. Individual Psychotherapy

Individual therapy with pediatric patients is frequently indicated as the result of a mental health consultation. In general, the same principles that apply to individual therapy with physically healthy children are relevant to the treatment of a child with a physical illness. A therapeutic alliance, a clear treatment plan, a contract with the child and the parent, privacy, confidentiality, and the power of the relationship are all essential components of psychotherapy with any patient. However, several additional factors are also crucial when the patient has a physical illness.

First, although the consultation paves the way for the introduction of psychological issues as germane to the management of the illness, the child and the family will not easily shift from a somatic to a psychological focus. When psychotherapy does not "take" with pediatric patients, it is often because the therapist uses psychological language, whereas the patient and the parents think and speak in terms of physical illness, medical problems, and somatic dysfunction. A therapist new to working with physically ill patients may try to confront this somatic disposition early in therapy in an attempt to deal with the "real" or "underlying" issues. At such times, the patient feels misunderstood and senses that the therapy will not be helpful.

A second component of successful individual therapy with

pediatric patients is respect. The therapist must respect the reality of the medical situation. Although intrapsychic factors are always relevant, mental health professionals are prone to underestimate or be less interested in the myriad realistic stressors associated with a chronic or potentially fatal illness. The therapist must also respect the patient's creativity in discovering individually appropriate coping solutions. Our definitions and standards for judging what constitutes "normal" development, appropriate defenses, and satisfactory mental health are all based on the behavior of physically healthy, able-bodied children. These definitions and standards apply only partially or not at all to children with a serious illness or physical handicap. Together, the therapist and patient must take a fresh look at what constitutes coping in this unique situation.

A third factor that bears emphasis in individual therapy with pediatric patients is the importance of ventilation in the context of an empathic relationship. The need to express strong feelings and to have them understood is powerful. For chronically ill children and adolescents, the limiting factor is often how much emotional expression others can tolerate. They may fear displeasing adults on whom they depend for their treatment, or they may seek to protect those they care for from the intensity of their feelings. Individual therapy may be a unique outlet for these children. Audiotapes, videotapes, journals, and drawings can be used to facilitate emotional expression in the context of therapy.

Finally, the issue of confidentiality may be troubling to the psychiatrist or psychologist working with a child who is also being treated by a pediatric team. Pediatricians need and deserve regular communication from therapists who treat their patients. The lack of such communication is a major criticism voiced by pediatricians about mental health professionals (Fritz and Bergman 1985). At the same time, individual therapy goes nowhere when confidentiality is not guaranteed. Mental health professionals must realize that the feedback pediatricians want almost never violates the spirit of confidentiality. Pediatricians need only general summaries of the progress of therapy and advice about how they can improve their management of the child based on the knowledge gained by the therapist from the individual work. Children understand and accept this degree of contact if they know that the personal details they disclose will remain confidential. Pediatricians, in turn, are spared the frustration of working totally in the dark, and their effectiveness in managing the child is greatly enhanced by brief but regular communication.

2. Cognitive-Behavior Interventions

There are a number of specific, symptom-focused cognitive and behavioral strategies that should be considered when devising interventions involving pediatric patients. These strategies are particularly useful in the pediatric setting and are described in some detail in the following sections because of their relevance to consultants.

a. Contingency management

When a consultant is asked to make recommendations on how best to increase or decrease certain behaviors of a hospitalized child, contingency management procedures should be considered. Examples of frequently needed behavioral changes include decreasing crying or disruptive behavior, increasing compliance with medical regimens, decreasing refusal to take pills or cooperate with medical procedures, and increasing oral food intake in chronically ill children. *Reinforcement* of the desired behavior is almost always the first choice among the different treatments. For example, if a child in the intensive care unit refuses to take oral medications, a simple positive reinforcement, such as a sticker each time he or she takes a pill, should be tried first; if this reinforcement is successful, it can be maintained by either parents or nursing staff. The stickers then might be collected and traded for prizes of various sizes. If the program fails to alter the behavior, the consultant should consider whether the reinforcer is powerful enough or whether other reinforcers (e.g., attention paid to the patient by parents when he or she does not take the pill) override the reinforcement program. If the former is the problem, the solution is to provide better rewards. If the latter is the problem, one must remove the reinforcer (parental attention) that maintains the noncompliant behavior; this procedure is called *extinction*. The consultant might suggest that the parents leave the child's room and let the nurse oversee pill taking. By so doing, attention to all the negative behaviors associated with pill taking (i.e., fussing, whining, and pleading) is removed as long as the nurse remains neutral and does not reinforce these behaviors.

Punishment procedures in the hospital usually involve restricting the child's mobility (i.e., making the child stay in the room or limiting access to visitors). For example, if an adolescent with anorexia does not eat a certain prespecified amount of food at a meal, then the consequence is remaining in bed until the next meal. Similarly, access to the playroom can be contingent on the patient's compliance with prescribed medical treatment (e.g., chest physiotherapy in a child with cystic fibrosis). One particular variant of punishment, response cost, is sometimes more effective than other approaches. For example, a patient is given a certain amount of television-viewing time per day, but every time the patient does not make the desired response (e.g., performing personal hygiene tasks), he or she loses a specified amount of television-viewing time.

Contingency management approaches to treatment (i.e., the use of both positive reinforcement and punishment) are particularly applicable to young children as exemplified in the following case example:

Billy was a 2-year-old boy with severe atopic dermatitis. Constant, deep scratching led to superficial infection and worse itching. A week of baseline monitoring revealed that scratching was particularly bad at bedtime and often escalated after Billy was reprimanded by his parents or when he was bored. Billy's concerned, and usually quite competent, parents typically responded in the following sequence: asking Billy to stop scratching, trying to distract him from the scratching, and finally reprimanding him and giving him a spanking.

The first intervention involved instructing Billy's parents to pay less attention to him when he was scratching and to greatly increase the amount of attention they paid to him when he didn't scratch. For example, if Billy began to scratch when his parents were playing with him, they were instructed to turn their heads away until Billy stopped scratching (extinction). At that time, they were told to redirect their attention to Billy. In addition, the parents were told to praise (reinforce) Billy for scratch-free periods ("I really like it when you don't scratch your skin when we're playing"). At bedtime, it was necessary to rearrange the contingencies to get some control over the scratching. Billy's bedtime story was delayed until he demonstrated several minutes of not scratching. This time was gradually lengthened so that eventually Billy demonstrated a half-hour of not scratching in bed before he was read his bedtime story. This treatment approach used over a 6-week period resulted in almost complete cessation of scratching.

Contracts are intervention techniques that often add to the power of behavioral programs. In a *behavioral contract,* a specific behavior is defined and the consequences of performing that behavior are clearly outlined. Contracts are put in writing, and the behaviors to be performed by all parties are well specified. For example, for a child who is noncompliant with medications, a contract might read as follows:

Responsibilities	Privileges
1. Bob will take his daily medications within 10 minutes of being requested to do so by parents.	1. Bob will be allowed 10 minutes of additional TV-viewing time per day.

Bonus: If Bob successfully takes all his pills within 10 minutes 80% of the time over 1 week, his parents agree to let Bob invite a friend to sleep over on Saturday night.

Sanction: If Bob fails to take his pills within 10 minutes, the extra TV-viewing time privilege will be withheld. If failure occurs three or more times within 2 days, he will lose 1 hour of TV time until he takes all medications on time for 2 straight days.

Contracts are often particularly useful when negotiating parent-adolescent conflict related to the medical regimen. A detailed description of behavioral contracting for a child with cystic fibrosis has been described by Stark et al. (1987).

b. Relaxation training

Relaxation training is a rather simple technique that has been shown to be effective in patients with a number of somatic disorders such as headaches, recurrent abdominal pain, mildly elevated heart rate, various sleep disturbances including insomnia, and treatment of medically related fears and phobias. Many different types of relaxation have been described, including progressive muscle relaxation, mental imagery, and autogenics (for an overview, see Powers and Spirito, in press).

To maximize the effectiveness of relaxation, the patient's preferred technique for relaxing should be assessed. Such an assessment should indicate whether imagery is more desirable than progressive muscle relaxation, as well as which words and phrases the individual child uses to describe feelings of relaxation. One effective approach to relaxation is first to teach the patient deep muscle relaxation and then to use imagery to enhance and maintain the relaxed sensation. Slow, deep breathing throughout such training usually is also helpful. In most cases, especially in the hospital, it is preferable to audiotape the session so the patient can listen to the relaxation exercise as needed. By using a tape, the patient is able to avoid many of the outside distractions that occur on a hospital floor. The audiotape can be modified as needed in follow-up consultation visits to maximize the effectiveness of the training. Relaxation training can be useful even in children with terminal illness, as the following case example illustrates:

Beth, a 17-year-old girl with end-stage cystic fibrosis, was referred because of hyperventilation episodes and sleep difficulties. An evaluation concluded that extreme anxiety about her health status (chronic mucus congestion, pneumonia, and severely compromised lung function) was exacerbating her sleep difficulties. Beth's labored breathing provided a cue (inappropriate stimulus) for anxiety rather than an adaptive coping response. Despite her significant pulmonary problems, Beth was taught a meditative breathing procedure to help her relax. During meditative breathing, she was asked to take occasional deep breaths, hold them, and let them out. An autogenic phrase (i.e., a statement Beth made to herself to help enhance the feelings of relaxation) was added. In Beth's case, "calm" was sufficient to enhance the efficacy of the relaxation procedure. In addition, a simple adaptive coping statement, "Don't panic, just relax," was taught to Beth to help circumvent the onset of hyperventilation when Beth's breathing became particularly labored. An audiotape was made of the technique so Beth was able to practice during the hospitalization despite the frequent commotion and noises on the ward. Although the meditative procedure was somewhat helpful, Beth also reported significant muscle tension in her shoulders because she was constantly sitting to breathe more comfortably. Thus, a progressive muscle relaxation exercise focusing on this muscle group was added to the relaxation procedure. Beth used this exercise in conjunction with the autogenics and meditative breathing to derive considerable relief in the last months of her life.

c. **Biofeedback training**

Biofeedback can be defined as the use of sensitive monitoring equipment to provide an individual with information about a physiological parameter that he or she is not usually aware of, so that the physiological function can be modified. Typical biofeedback equipment, whether it is computer based or free-standing, provides the patient with some continuous visual or auditory feedback about target parameters. Portable equipment is available for use on inpatient ward consultations. The concept of biofeedback seems to be reasonably well understood by children as young as age 7. (For a review of the use of biofeedback in general, see Schwartz et al. 1987 and Spirito and Powers, in press; for a review of its use for certain focused symptoms, see Varni 1983.)

Biofeedback is often used as a means of enhancing the effects of relaxation training or desensitization. In such cases, electrodes are typically placed on the forehead to measure frontalis electromyograph activity and on the finger to measure peripheral finger temperature. The placement of electrodes in these areas is explained to the child as a way to measure muscle tension and blood flow, two indicators of the amount of stress that the body is experiencing. A very simple explanation is used (e.g., when the body is under stress, muscles become tense and blood flow slows down). It is important to explain that temperature is an indirect way to measure blood flow; the more the blood flow, the higher the finger temperature.

Biofeedback is often used with childhood headache patients. If the child describes a bifrontal location of the headache pain, then using electromyograph frontalis placement to measure muscle activity in the forehead is very easily understood by the child as a way to treat headaches. If the child has migraine headaches, the suspected relationship between blood flow and migraine headaches can be explained to the child in his or her own language. Peripheral temperature training can be explained as a way of teaching the child to get better control over blood flow, which in turn will affect headaches. (For more detailed examples of the clinical usefulness of biofeedback training with both adults and children, see Blanchard and Andrasik 1985.) Biofeedback training may also be recommended as a major treatment approach for specific conditions such as Raynaud's syndrome, mild hypertension, urinary or fecal incontinence, and certain neuromuscular disorders such as spasmodic torticollis.

d. Systematic desensitization

Medically related fears (e.g., fear of computed tomography scans) or conditioned responses (e.g., anticipatory nausea and vomiting in chemotherapy patients) may require more concerted efforts than simple relaxation training for a successful outcome. In such cases, anxiety is precipitated primarily by either antecedent stimuli in the environment, such as the events leading up to insertion of an intravenous line, or the patient's own cognitions. In a desensitization approach, the patient is first taught relaxation and some cognitive statements to help lower the arousal. Then, he or she is gradually exposed to the feared stimuli, either in imagination or by direct contact with the stimulus, according to a hierarchy of feared events prepared by the patient. For example, for a bone marrow aspiration, the patient is asked to outline the steps leading up to the procedure: walking to the treatment room, lying down on the table, assuming a curled position, and so on. The patient is then exposed to the situation, either directly or in his or her imagination. In the case of extreme fears, it may be most helpful to begin desensitization in imagination before progressing to in vivo desensitization. For most hospital-related fears, direct exposure is preferred. The patient is presented with each step in the hierarchy until he or she is able to master the anxiety and maintain a relatively relaxed state. At that point, the next scene or circumstance in the hierarchy is presented until the patient no longer feels anxious. The following case example illustrates the use of in vivo systematic desensitization for a medically related fear:

Mark, an 11-year-old boy, was referred by a neurologist because of fainting spells that occurred secondary to a vasovagal episode after extreme fear. The child's fear was associated with medically related stimuli, including the sight of a sick or handicapped person. For example, on one occasion at school, Mark fainted after viewing a movie on handicapped children. On another occasion, Mark fainted when he heard his parents talking about his grandfather, who had recently had his leg amputated because of diabetes. Mark was trained in simple ways of relaxing and in the use of positive self-statements to counter his negative cognition about handicapped people and medically related fears. Self-statements about medical fears (e.g., "Stay calm, relax," "There's nothing that can hurt me, just take a deep breath and relax," "There's no need to get upset: people with handicaps are just the same as me") were derived after interviewing Mark about the cognitive basis for his fears. Four outpatient sessions of in vivo desensitization were then conducted. Permission was obtained from nursing staff for the child to walk through inpatient pediatric floors. Mark was gradually exposed to children who looked "normal" except for an intravenous line inserted in their hand, children in casts of various sorts, and to a child who was intubated. As he demonstrated that he was able to master his anxiety with each more-threatening medical condition, Mark was praised and then exposed to the next more-threatening problem. If he became too nervous when exposed to a patient, Mark stepped away, took a deep breath, reviewed the cognitive self-statements with the therapist, and then tried again when he felt ready. By using this approach over four sessions, Mark was able to master all experiences in the hospital with relatively little anxiety. To ensure that this treatment was generalized outside the hospital, the therapist recommended that the parents rent various movies that contained different medical themes and watch them with Mark. A 2-year follow-up revealed no further incidents of fainting.

e. Hypnotherapy

Hypnotherapy is often a potent treatment approach in the pediatric setting. Hypnosis refers to an altered state of consciousness that develops after inducing a state of deep relaxation. In such a deeply relaxed state, the patient is open to suggestion, which can then lead to behavior change. Hypnotherapy differs from hypnosis in that once the hypnotic state is entered, therapeutic interventions are delivered either by the patients themselves through self-hypnosis or by the therapist (Gardner and Olness 1981). When suggesting hypnotherapy as a treatment approach, the therapist should explain that hypnotherapy is a medical procedure and different from the types of hypnosis patients may have been exposed to in the media. The treatment approach will not be effective unless misconceptions and fears about hypnosis are allayed. Hypnotherapy has been used for many different symptoms, such as helping pediatric cancer patients deal with pain and distress encountered during invasive medical procedures. An excellent overview of the different applications of hypnosis and the induction techniques and suggestions that are useful with children can be found in Gardner and Olness (1981). The following case example illustrates the use of hypnotherapy for a patient with a somatic complaint:

Mary, an 11-year-old girl with a history of many different psychosomatic complaints, developed a pattern of sneezing approximately every 5 seconds. This sneezing persisted for a 6-week period, stopped when she was asleep, and kept her from attending school. Mary was seen by an allergist who attempted a number of different treatments, including the use of steroids, without success. She was subsequently referred to a child psychiatry program where hypnotherapy was recommended as the initial treatment for the debilitating symptom.

A clear rationale for the use of hypnotherapy was established to ensure the success of this technique. The sneezing reflex was discussed with Mary, and an analogy was made to having a switch in her head that somehow got stuck in the "on" position. Because no medicines or other techniques such as inserting a needle into the brain could turn off the sneeze center, hypnotherapy was used. After an entire session was spent describing the rationale for the procedure and details about hypnotherapy, a second session was scheduled in which an eye-roll hypnotic induction technique was used. Imagery-based procedures and deepening techniques induced a state of deep relaxation. Once Mary appeared deeply relaxed, a series of suggestions described how, during this hypnotic state, we would be able to talk directly to her unconscious mind to turn off the "sneeze center." She was asked to visualize the switch slowly moving towards the "off" position. The exact time when the sneezing would totally disappear was left ambiguous; it could be immediate or could take anywhere from several hours to several days. Mary responded favorably. The intensity of the sneeze decreased and the latency between sneezing increased significantly during the hypnotic procedure itself. An audiotape of the procedure enabled Mary to practice at home on a daily basis. Over the course of the next 5 days, the sneezing gradually diminished. After 6 weeks of constant sneezing, the problem stopped completely.

3. Limitations of the Pediatric Setting

It is readily apparent to any mental health professional that a general pediatric floor is a very different place from a psychiatric ward. It is organized around an average length of stay of 3–5 days and a high level of physical impairment in patients. Privacy, quiet, and consistency are usually in short supply. House staff and medical students rotate on and off the service frequently and at different times. Nurses change shifts and patient assignments often. Even when a majority of the patients are exhibiting psychological disturbances, many staff see their role as narrowly limited to treating physical illness. Within this environment, the consultant psychiatrist or psychologist must consider the feasibility of a particular intervention carefully before suggesting it. For example, a reinforcement schedule or a behavioral contract that seems straightforward to the consultant may evoke resistance on an acute unit or overwhelm a busy, psychologically unsophisticated staff. Because of the turnover in physicians and nurses on a pediatric ward, a major teaching effort around a particular case may not necessarily mean that the same intervention can be more easily accomplished the next time. The experienced consultant is cautious about recommending psychological interventions that involve a sustained effort by the pediatric ward staff. Accumulated experience with a particular unit will help the consultant to judge what are realistic expectations.

4. Psychosomatic Inpatient Units

The consultant may encounter patients who need a level of psychological care that is beyond the capacity of the pediatric staff, even with considerable consultation. The most intensive psychological intervention is hospitalization in a pediatric psychosomatic unit, previously described in detail (Fritz et al. 1981). Such a service is designed for patients whose combined medical and psychological symptoms are refractory to outpatient interventions and whose development and general functioning are disrupted by the disorders. The staff on an acute pediatric ward usually have neither the time nor the training to deal with the psychological complexities these cases present, whereas most psychiatric wards lack the capacity to provide the acute medical care needed to manage significant medical problems.

The psychosomatic inpatient unit therefore serves a critical function for children with severe combined pediatric and psychiatric problems. Fortunately, such units are becoming increasingly common in modern children's hospitals and are available to many patients close enough to home to permit regular family involvement. Treatment typically entails daily group and individual therapy, a highly structured milieu that incorporates many of the behavior modification approaches described above, and at least weekly family sessions. The specific goals and therapeutic strategies are individually tailored. Close communication between pediatricians and the treatment team is assiduously maintained. When a psychosomatic unit is available for appropriate patients, the most comprehensive, integrated pediatric and psychiatric care can be provided. Such units provide a much needed element in the range of interventions available to the pediatric mental health consultant and have proven to be both clinically effective and cost-effective.

5. Referral to Traditional Psychiatric Ward

Some patients who are hospitalized acutely on a pediatric ward will need to be transferred to a traditional child and adolescent psychiatric inpatient unit. In areas where a psychosomatic unit is not available, the traditional psychiatric ward is the only alternative. The consultant should help arrange necessary pediatric follow-up to the psychiatric unit on which the patient is being hospitalized, because frequently subspecialty pediatric care is not routinely available on traditional units. The consultant serves to bridge the gap between pediatrics and psychiatry for the particular case, even when formal programmatic changes are not desired or possible.

Referral to a traditional psychiatric ward rather than a psychosomatic unit is also appropriate when the patient's psychopathology or behavior exceeds that with which a psychosomatic program is prepared to deal. Frequently, a psychosomatic unit is established on a converted pediatric ward and thus lacks locked-unit capacity; seclusion rooms; suicide-safe shower rods, closets, and so forth; bolted-down beds for restraint; shatterproof glass; and other features common on well-designed psychiatric wards. Patients who are psychotic, actively suicidal, extremely violent, or likely to run away need the full resources of a traditional psychiatric ward even if significant pediatric illness complicates the picture. Providing coordinated care on a psychiatric ward for a severely disturbed child or adolescent who also has a serious physical illness presents a major challenge to all involved; fortunately, it is a relatively uncommon circumstance.

E. REFERENCES

Blanchard EB, Andrasik F: Management of Chronic Headaches: A Psychological Approach. New York, Pergamon, 1985

Bronheim S, Jacobstein DM: Psychosocial assessment in chronic and fatal illness, in Psychological and Behavioral Assessment: Impact on Pediatric Care. Edited by Magrab PR. New York, Plenum, 1984, pp 279–336

Drigan R, Spirito A, Gelber RD: Behavioral effects of corticosteroids in children with acute lymphoblastic leukemia. Med Pediatr Oncol 20:13–21, 1992

Fritz GK: Psychological issues in assessing and managing asthma in children. Clin Rev Allergy 5:259–271,1987

Fritz GK: Child psychiatry consultation-liaison and the evolution of pediatric psychiatry. Psychosomatics 31:85–90, 1990

Fritz GK, Bergman AS: Child psychiatrists through pediatricians' eyes: results of a national survey. J Am Acad Child Adolesc Psychiatry 24:81–86, 1985

Fritz GK, Steiner H, Hilliard J, et al: Pediatric and psychiatric collaboration in the management of childhood asthma. Clin Pediatr (Phila) 20:772–776, 1981

Gardner G, Olness K: Hypnosis and Hypnotherapy With Children. New York, Grune & Stratton, 1981

Harris JC, Carel CA, Rosenberg LA, et al: Intermittent high dose corticosteroid treatment in childhood cancer: behavioral and emotional consequences. J Am Acad Child Adolesc Psychiatry 25:120–124, 1986

Ling MHM, Perry PJ, Tsuang MT: Side effects of corticosteroid therapy: psychiatry aspects. Arch Gen Psychiatry 38:471–477, 1981

Lobato D: Brothers, Sisters, and Special Needs. Baltimore, MD, Paul H. Brooks Publishing, 1990

Magrab PR: Psychosocial development of chronically ill children, in Issues in the Care of Children With Chronic Illness. Edited by Hobbs N, Perrin JM. San Francisco, Jossey- Bass, 1985, pp 698–715

Powers S, Spirito A: Relaxation, in Handbook of Child and Adolescent Psychiatry. Edited by Eth S, Harrison S. New York, Wiley (in press)

Schecter NL: Pain and pain control in children. Curr Probl Pediatr 15:1–67, 1985

Schwartz M, and associates: Biofeedback: A Practitioner's Guide. New York, Guilford, 1987

Spirito A, Powers S: Biofeedback, in Handbook of Child and Adolescent Psychiatry. Edited by Eth S, Harrison S. New York, Wiley (in press)

Stark LJ, Miller ST, Plienes AJ, et al: Behavioral contracting to increase chest physiotherapy: a study of a young cystic fibrosis patient. Behav Modif 11:75–86, 1987

Varni J: Clinical Behavioral Pediatrics. New York, Pergamon, 1983

Willis DJ, Elliott CH, Jay SM: Psychological effects of physical illness and its concomitants, in Handbook for the Practice of Pediatric Psychology. Edited by Tuma J. New York, Wiley, 1982, pp 28–66

SCHOOL CONSULTATION

Richard E. Mattison, M.D.
Anthony Spirito, Ph.D.

Section II: School Consultation

Chapter Five
Consultation in the School Environment
  A. Psychological skills of school staff
  B. Special classes
    1. SED resource room
    2. Self-contained SED classroom in a regular school
    3. SED school
  C. SED students
    1. Identification
    2. Characteristics
    3. Outcome
  D. What school staff needs from consulting child
     psychiatrists and psychologists
  E. References

Chapter Six
A Model for SED Case Evaluation
  A. Overview of the model
  B. Review of referral information
    1. School psychologist evaluation
    2. Previous evaluations
    3. Teacher behavior checklist
    4. Parent behavior checklist
  C. Initial meeting with multidisciplinary team
  D. Student interview
  E. Parent interview
  F. Feedback to team and collaborative treatment planning
  G. Feedback to parent(s) and student
  H. Report preparation
  I. Summary
  J. References

Chapter Seven
Principles in Common School Case Consultations
  A. Elementary school (case 1)
  B. Junior high school (case 2)

CHAPTER FIVE

Consultation in the School Environment

Richard E. Mattison, M.D.

In terms of the needs of students with psychiatric illness, today's schools have improved; however, they are still designed primarily for the average student. Educators are more knowledgeable about child and adolescent development, more aware of mental health issues in school, and better trained in individual, behavioral, and group management. However, their expertise can best address pupils' problems in adjusting to the school environment, the common stresses affecting children or teenagers, and the symptoms of mild psychiatric disorders. As a pupil's problems become more severe, the school staff's capacity to handle such problems is soon exceeded. Then, more specialized school intervention should occur, ideally with consultation by a child psychologist or psychiatrist.

Educators and child mental health professionals have historically had a tenuous relationship. Both disciplines have limited training for collaboration, and time demands often preclude face-to-face interaction. Different technical languages have been spoken; for example, educators have been and continue to be behaviorally oriented, whereas child psychiatrists quite frequently have been psychodynamically minded, especially in the past. Thus, communication (when it occurred) was commonly strained, and in the subsequent frustration, school staff handled children one way in school and the psychiatrists or psychologists treated them in another manner in the office. Mutual unfamiliarity and premature dismissal of the usefulness of another discipline are still common.

Current conditions are promoting better working relationships between educators and child mental health consultants. The lay public is becoming better educated about psychiatric illness and consequently are demanding more response from educators for children who need intervention. The need for multimodality intervention (including educational interventions) for the disorders of so many students has become more recognized by child psychiatrists and psychologists. However, constraints of time, finances, and training continue to preclude as much collaboration as would be desirable.

Possibly most reflective of the relationship between the disciplines is the rarity of collaborative research. For example, child psychiatrists seldom publish in educational journals. Similarly, few articles addressing school issues appear in child psychiatry journals. This problem is further reflected by research design. Educators study the progress of students in school but rarely simultaneously investigate change at home or indicate what outside intervention was also used. The same can be said of research by child psychiatrists. Whereas psychiatric studies often assess change in the school with behavior checklists, they rarely specify what intervention was done at school, if indeed any controlled treatment was designed for the classroom. To remedy this collaboration problem, not only for the sake of students with psychiatric disorders but also to stimulate mutual research projects, educators and child mental health consultants must continue to attempt to understand each other's disciplines and to improve collaborative efforts.

This brief introduction serves as an overview of the current relationship between educators and child mental health professionals. To promote better consultation work in schools, Chapters 5–8 have been written for child psychiatrists and psychologists. This chapter describes the typical school environment for students with psychiatric disorders. It focuses on the psychological skills and limitations of school staff from the different educational disciplines. Special classes for children and teenagers with severe psychiatric disorders are discussed. Finally, general needs of school staffs that can be addressed by child psychologists and psychiatrists are outlined.

A. PSYCHOLOGICAL SKILLS OF SCHOOL STAFF

When a child psychiatrist or psychologist begins to work with a new school staff in the care of a pupil, he or she should meet all the personnel who could have a role in managing the child: teacher(s), the principal (or assistant principal), the guidance counselor, and the school psychologist. The clinician must determine what strengths and limitations each staff member brings to the task of doing psychological work with the student.

Generally, the above school staff (excluding school psychologists) have certain characteristics in common. They have limited knowledge of DSM-III-R diagnoses (American Psychiatric Association 1987) and of the accrued knowledge in child psychiatry for each diagnostic category. Their management skills (behavioral, group, or individual) may be sufficient for pupils with minor problems, but may be insufficient for pupils with more severe difficulties. Educational personnel have limited training in dealing with families, especially regarding emotional situations. In addition, their working knowledge of a student's family may be incomplete, anecdotal, or dangerously piecemeal. Finally, far too many school staff members have done little work with any child mental health professional.

Of all the school staff, *teachers* have the best overall knowledge of a student, and the breadth of their information should not be overlooked. They are generally aware of a great deal more than a student's cognitive status and classroom behavioral problems. The range of their potentially valuable information includes the pupil's assets, moods, social skills and weaknesses, after-school or neighborhood activities, and family. Teachers also can offer observations about their experiences with the parent(s) and past or current family history and stressors, although one must be cautious when weighing such information. Teachers may already have a working relationship with the family. Despite their limited psychological training, the therapeutic potential and ingenuity of teachers should not be underestimated. Indeed, their understanding of a student's problems and present treatment should always be ascertained. Furthermore, despite the multiple demands on teachers' time, they are often willing to devote increased effort toward a particular child, as long as they receive clear recommendations and continuing support.

However, teachers can get overwhelmed by all they have to know, do, and fill out for their job, and childhood and adolescent psychiatric disorders are not at the top of the list. Consequently, teachers all too often have to manage dysfunctional students without sufficient training about their disorders or treatment (Zabel 1988). Given limited administrative response or support, a teacher does the best he or she can, based on the self-generated hypothesis that drives his or her interaction with a student. This relationship can become a powerful determinant, good or bad, in a pupil's educational career; if the relationship is negative, it will be difficult to overcome later. Negative interaction is especially likely to occur if a teacher resents the extra time it takes to work with a student who has a behavior problem.

Guidance counselors are often the first school staff members to whom teachers reach out for assistance. They are frequently teachers who have obtained master's degree training in guidance counseling. Counselors can assess the student more extensively, including meeting with the parent(s). They also have more training (although, again, the training is quite variable) in individual counseling and group work, and they are more aware of community mental health resources. They may be trained to provide specialized therapeutic intervention (e.g., group therapy for students whose parents are divorcing or for children with limited social skills).

However, guidance counselors are usually responsible for large numbers of children and thus can spend a limited amount of time with individual children. In high school, they may primarily focus on postgraduation planning. Although they are often called on to determine whether a child is psychologically disturbed, they are often frustrated by their limited training for this responsibility. Similarly, they are often asked to advise a teacher on proper classroom intervention, but their knowledge in this area can also be limited.

The next internal resource for assistance is the *school psychologist*. School psychologists have more extensive training in the evaluation and care of students with psychiatric disorders, and they commonly have master's degrees. Their knowledge of DSM-III-R disordersmay be considerable, and their therapeutic skills, especially in behavioral modification, enable them to greatly assist in classroom management.

Generally, the primary assignment of school psychologists is cognitive testing of pupils, again with the responsibility for large numbers of pupils in different schools. Thus the time they have available for dysfunctional students with psychiatric difficulties is generally limited, or they are available only for evaluation rather than leading the school team in the care of such students. Frequently, skills that were well developed after their own training have deteriorated from disuse or become outdated because of limited time for reeducation.

Finally, *school principals or assistant principals* may have gained knowledge about students with psychiatric difficulties during their teaching careers. This experience can be invaluable, especially when they interact with or lead school teams that often exist to review and plan for problematic students. Importantly, the power of the principals' position can often move a case along, especially with regard to convincing a family to seek outside help.

In contrast, if a principal has a pessimistic or hostile attitude toward students with psychiatric disorders, the identification and care of these children can be impeded or disrupted. Proper referrals can be discouraged, or staff may not be encouraged to devote the extra time necessary for such students. Furthermore, preventive mental health measures and appropriate school services may not be sufficiently developed.

Finally, the nature of the teacher-student relationship at the different educational levels (e.g., elementary versus secondary school) is a powerful factor. In grade school, a student has one teacher who knows him or her very well, which allows the intervention to be more focused and coordinated. Academic and social demands on students in grade school also are somewhat more manageable. These demands rapidly expand in secondary school, as do the number of staff involved with a student. Coordinating several teachers to use the same approach with a pupil can be more difficult. Thus, the secondary school student with psychopathology generally must survive in less accommodating, less flexible circumstances.

B. SPECIAL CLASSES

Depending on his or her ability, a teacher may be able to address a child's psychological difficulties in a regular classroom. Or the guidance counselor may be able to provide additional assistance that will enable a student to remain in regular programming: individual counseling once or twice a week, group work specific to the student's difficulties, or referral of the family for outside intervention to complement the help in school. Finally, the school psychologist may be able to help the student remain in the same classroom (e.g., by providing individualized behavioral planning that the teacher can use with the psychologist's support).

However, when these steps prove insufficient, then the student with more serious psychopathology must be referred by the principal for evaluation for special education. Special education can be delivered in any of the settings described below (the setting usually depends on the severity of the dysfunction). These students receive a variety of labels, such as behaviorally disordered, emotionally handicapped, and seriously emotionally disturbed (SED). The latter abbreviation, SED, is used here generically for students who require special school intervention for their serious behavioral or emotional disorders (excluding only autism).

When a student is referred for evaluation for placement in an SED setting, he or she then enters a separate special-education administrative structure. A multidisciplinary diagnostic team from the special-education program assesses the student's history and the school's past interventions, as well as testing and interviewing the child. History from the parent(s) is also obtained. Once the child is accepted as an SED student, services become available from the special-education program's teachers, psychologists, and social workers, who are skilled at working with SED students. A specific individualized education plan (IEP) is then developed with parental approval to address the varied needs of each student; this plan can be implemented in the different settings described below.

1. SED Resource Room

Often a student will need intervention that is more specialized or more intensive than can be provided in a regular classroom, but that still allows him or her to remain primarily in regular classes. Daily classes in a resource room with a special-education teacher who has had SED training may suffice. In such a setting, the teacher can provide cognitive-behavioral intervention, more intensive individual counseling, or group work. The setting may also provide relief and encouragement so that the student can maintain more consistent functioning in regular classes. Furthermore, the SED resource room teacher may be able to consult with the other regular classroom teachers to coordinate a single plan implemented by all staff for a child. Such daily special classes may be especially helpful to students whose functioning is starting to deteriorate in a regular classroom or who are making the transition from a more intensive special-education setting or from psychiatric hospitalization.

One limitation of a resource room is the large number of students who may rotate through the setting each day (e.g., 30–50), presenting quite a challenge to the teacher. It can be difficult for the resource room teacher to keep pace with all the students' individual needs and to find time to consult with each child's teachers. Also, resource rooms may in fact contain mixes of students with psychiatric disorders, learning disabilities, and even mild mental retardation. In addition, although the teacher is certified to teach children with different special-education needs, he or she may have primary expertise in areas other than SED.

2. Self-contained SED Classroom in a Regular School

The SED classroom in a regular school contains approximately 10 students, all with the SED designation, and the majority of a student's school day is spent in this classroom. An SED teacher and often a trained aide are available to intensively focus on the students' difficulties, individually and in groups. SED teachers' training and experience generally focus primarily on SED students, and they can more comfortably and adeptly collaborate with community mental health resources. Generally, SED classrooms have a behavioral modification plan that applies to everyone, with individualized tailoring according to each student's needs.

A common problem for self-contained SED classrooms is the lack of support services. That is, if a student's condition is severe enough to require intervention at this level, such a student also requires further intervention by a community resource, and most likely the family needs help as well. Too frequently, such community treatment is not available; the SED teacher may not have any assistance in finding the necessary outside help for the child and family; or the family may resist referral. Thus, without comprehensive treatment, the progress of the student may be limited.

3. SED School

A separate SED school (often a small, converted public school) is dedicated just to SED students for whom less-intensive SED intervention has not succeeded or who need immediate intervention at this level. In this setting, additional professionals are available to assist the SED teachers and the students. They may include a principal, who is often a master SED teacher; a social worker who deals with family problems and crises and coordinates community services; and a school psychologist whose time is devoted primarily to therapeutic intervention with the students in that special school.

The greater number of staff members allows more effort to be applied to finding community resources and to collaborating with outside professionals. In such a conducive setting, community therapists will often come to the school. The additional staff are also available to assist teachers when crises arise or on particularly bad days.

However, certain problems are often associated with this level of intervention. Students's problems may be serious enough to require residential placement or a probational facility, but the family or community resources may be insufficient. Then, the SED school must bear the brunt of providing services. If there are too many severely disturbed students in an SED school, the staff will be overwhelmed, to the detriment of all the pupils. On the other hand, it is often difficult for SED students from an SED school to return to a regular school environment. They may greatly miss the intensive support system. Or transitional assistance—which is especially important to ensure that the new school staff understand the student's needs, strengths, and weaknesses—may be lacking. Optimally, transitional staff should remain available to the new school staff and the student until the transition is complete.

C. SED STUDENTS

Of all children and teenagers in school, SED students are the ones most in need of attention by child psychiatrists and psychologists. Their problems are serious and complex, and most frequently the expertise of a child psychiatrist or psychologist is required to design and/or direct the multidisciplinary treatment of these students. This section provides some basic information to further familiarize child psychiatrists and psychologists with SED students.

1. Identification

The criteria necessary for SED classification were established by Public Law 94-142. At least one of the following five conditions has to exist "over a long period of time and to a marked degree, which adversely affects education performance":

1. An inability to learn which cannot be explained by intellectual, sensory, or health factors
2. An inability to build or maintain satisfactory interpersonal relationships with peers or teachers
3. Inappropriate types of behavior or feelings under normal circumstances
4. A general pervasive mood of unhappiness or depression
5. A tendency to develop physical symptoms or fears associated with personal or school problems

These criteria have been criticized by educators as vague and imprecise (Smith et al. 1988). The result has been much latitude in interpretation, most likely to the detriment of numerous needy students. Although the national average percentage of SED students served was 0.57% of all students in 1986–1987 (U.S. Department of Education 1988), many special educators feel the actual need is closer to 2%–3% (Morse 1985).

Because of this disappointment with the SED criteria, more precise criteria are being developed by the National Mental Health and Special Education Coalition. One member of this coalition, the Council for Children with Behavioral Disorders (1991), proposed the following criteria:

1. *Emotional or behavioral disorder* (*EBD*; a new term for SED) refers to a condition in which behavioral or emotional responses of an individual in school are so different from his or her generally accepted, age-appropriate, ethnic, or cultural norms that they adversely affect educational performance in such areas as self-care, social relationships, personal adjustment, academic progress, classroom behavior, or work adjustment.
2. EBD is more than a transient, expected response to stressors in the child's or youth's environment and would persist even with individualized interventions, such as feedback to the individual, consultation with parents or families, and modifications of the educational environment.
3. The eligibility decision must be based on multiple sources of data about the individual's behavioral or emotional functioning. EBD must be exhibited in at least two different settings, at least one of which is school-related.
4. EBD can coexist with other handicapping conditions, as defined elsewhere in this law.
5. This category may include children or youths with schizophrenia, affective disorders, anxiety disorders, or other sustained disturbances of conduct, attention, or adjustment.

Consultants who help multidisciplinary school teams evaluate students for SED class placement must obviously be familiar with these evolving criteria. Furthermore, a current criterion issue is causing much controversy: whether "socially maladjusted" students (i.e., primarily pupils with conduct disorders) should be excluded from classification as SED. An extensive discussion of this debate is presented in a special issue of *Behavioral Disorders* (Volume 15, No. 3, 1990).

2. Characteristics

Ideally, the development of new criteria would incorporate existing knowledge about the characteristics of SED students. Unfortunately, such basic information is quite sparse in both the educational and the child psychiatric literature. However, recent studies have begun to add some clarification (Mattison et al. 1986). Among both elementary and secondary students recommended for SED placement, boys predominated and an average level of intelligence was found. Too often, repeating a grade was the primary educational intervention, whereas only small percentages of students received any community psychological intervention at the time of recommendation for SED classes. Multiple family stressors were very common, particularly physical abuse and parental psychiatric illness. Although externalizing psychiatric disorders were the most common, a wide range of psychiatric diagnoses was found, as well as multiple diagnoses. Attention deficit disorder was identified in a majority of the elementary SED students, and depressive disorders were identified in a majority of the secondary SED students. Overall, the type of diagnosis did not appear to be as important as the severity of the illness for SED classification.

Thus more objective information about the characteristics of SED students is accruing. However, studies employing modern methodology remain necessary to further clarify characteristics of SED students and thereby assist future revisions of SED criteria.

3. Outcome

The outcome of SED students is essentially unknown, except that among all handicapped students aged 16–21 years who "exit" school, SED pupils typically show the highest dropout rate: 40.7% in 1985–1986 (U.S. Department of Education 1988).

Morse (1985) speculated that the prognosis of an SED student improves with higher IQ and socioeconomic status, younger age, and external support. However, forms of effective intervention and prognostic factors remain to be defined (Tindal 1985). Although we are beginning to learn the effects of different treatments on specific child psychiatric disorders, the next steps should include research into the impact of successful treatments on SED students with the target disorders and research into the usefulness of SED programming as a conjoint therapeutic modality.

D. WHAT SCHOOL STAFF NEED FROM CONSULTING CHILD PSYCHIATRISTS AND PSYCHOLOGISTS

The background material presented in this chapter begins to indicate what services school staffs need from consulting child psychiatrists and psychologists. When students demonstrate serious dysfunction in school, educators need increased understanding in terms of diagnosis and treatment planning. Their intervention roles need to be defined in practical terms. Their enhanced understanding should include more knowledge of the family in order to place the student in the context of environmental stresses, past and present. Frequently, feedback to the family is best coordinated by a child psychiatrist or psychologist who can thoroughly explain the diagnosis and treatment plan and answer associated questions. This interaction can in turn engage the family in a working, rather than an adversarial, relationship with the school staff and can direct the family to community resources, which are generally necessary as part of the comprehensive treatment plan.

Finally, pediatricians or family practitioners are frequently part of the overall intervention strategy; they prescribe medication or work with the family to provide a proper referral. Communication with physicians is much easier for a child mental health professional. Similarly, the initial communication with a current or future community therapist may be done more effectively by a child psychiatrist or psychologist than by one of the school staff.

At the systems level, collaborative interaction is the keystone. Child mental health professionals and educators both must continually educate each other about the current state of knowledge in their respective fields regarding children and teenagers with behavior and mood dysfunction in school. As a result, treatment needs and roles will become further clarified; in turn, this clarification will lead to revised training programs. Simultaneously, the need for collaborative research will also become clearer.

This summary of what schools need from consulting child psychiatrists and psychologists has been general, based on the primary focus of this chapter—an overview of the school environment. The next three chapters present specific information about case and systems consultations and continue to point out the realities of the school environment with which child mental health consultants must deal.

E. REFERENCES

American Psychiatric Association: Diagnostic and Statistical Manual of Mental Disorders, 3rd Edition, Revised. Washington, DC, American Psychiatric Association, 1987

Council for Children with Behavioral Disorders: New definition passes another hurdle. CCBD Newsletter, February 1, 1991, p 1

Mattison RE, Humphrey FJ, Kales SN, et al: Psychiatric background and diagnoses of children evaluated for special class placement. J Am Acad Child Psychiatry 25:514–520, 1986

Morse WC: The Education and Treatment of Socioemotionally Impaired Children and Youth. Syracuse, NY, Syracuse University Press, 1985

Smith CR, Wood FH, Grimes J: Issues in the identification and placement of behaviorally disordered students, in Handbook of Special Education: Research and Practice, Vol 2: Mildly Handicapped Conditions. Edited by Wang MC, Reynolds MC, Walberg HJ. New York, Pergamon Press, 1988, pp 95–123

Tindal G: Investigating the effectiveness of special education: an analysis of methodology. Journal of Learning Disabilities 18:101–112, 1985

U.S. Department of Education: Tenth annual report to Congress on the implementation of the Education of the Handicapped Act. Washington, DC, U.S. Government Printing Office, 1988

Zabel RH: Preparation of teachers for behaviorally disordered students: a review of literature, in Handbook of Special Education: Research and Practice, Vol 2: Mildly Handicapped Conditions. Edited by Wang MC, Reynolds MC, Walberg HJ. New York, Pergamon Press, 1988, pp 171–193

CHAPTER SIX

A Model for SED
Case Evaluation

Richard E. Mattison, M.D.

lthough child psychiatrists are required to learn school consultation as part of their training, the curriculum is not specified and therefore is quite variable. Similarly, literature on teaching school consultation has been sparse and has provided primarily general and anecdotal guidance (Berkovitz and Seliger 1985; Berkowitz 1975; Jellinek 1990). Although such material often proves helpful, school consultation could benefit from greater standardization, leading to more consistent training, a basis for ongoing refinement, and more objective research.

To begin with, case evaluation needs to be formalized. Possibly the most important example is consultation to help determine whether a student requires seriously emotionally disturbed (SED) programming as part of his or her comprehensive treatment needs. This evaluation typically involves a student with serious dysfunction, complex symptomatology, and crucial family stressors or impairment. A child psychiatrist or psychologist is consulted to provide a comprehensive evaluation of the child and the family and subsequently to work with a multidisciplinary school team to develop a treatment plan.

This chapter focuses on the description of an SED case evaluation model that I have developed over the past decade. Educator colleagues have greatly influenced its refinement, particularly by suggesting ways to improve its practicality, informativeness, and economy for school personnel.

A. OVERVIEW OF THE MODEL

This SED case evaluation model consists of the following sequential steps (with approximate time requirements in parentheses):

1. Review of referral information (15 minutes)
2. Initial meeting with school multidisciplinary team (30 minutes)
3. Student interview (45 minutes)
4. Parent(s) interview (45 minutes)
5. Feedback to the team and collaborative treatment planning (30 minutes)
6. Feedback to parent(s) and student (15 minutes)
7. Report preparation (30 minutes)

This overall procedure is consistent with standard practices of child mental health professionals, which have been adapted for school consultation. Each step is described in this chapter, with particular attention to aspects that are unique to school. The time requirements can vary, but 3 1/2 hours per consultation is a reasonable total time for fee negotiations with schools. Fees should be kept reasonable as reimbursement is 100%; a special-education program may be the most desirable agency with which to establish a contract. Potential advantages are a regular weekly time block, consistent multidisciplinary staff, the enhanced possibility of comprehensive treatment planning, and an ongoing working relationship that will foster trust, respect, and favorable impact on the care of SED students.

A practical problem throughout the evaluation is the organization and integration of all the information generated by the consultant. Also, questions and hypotheses that must be remembered and investigated continually arise. A working outline is suggested in Table 6–1. Such a worksheet allows the psychiatrist or psychologist to make ongoing important notes throughout the evaluation process, thus enhancing the building of knowledge toward a final diagnostic formulation. The worksheet also facilitates the final report preparation by enabling the consultant to collect and organize the condensed findings.

B. REVIEW OF REFERRAL INFORMATION

1. School Psychologist Evaluation

Many parts of the standard testing done by a school psychologist can help a consultant. The educational history of the student is vitally important to understand the chronology of the difficulties. The most useful school psychologist reports identify past and present staff observations of the student, as well as summarizing previous evaluations and interventions in the school environment. Information on the mental state of the student during the psychoeducational testing by the school psychologist is very useful to the consultant for comparison with the mental state during the consultation interview.

Intelligence and achievement tests are the standard core of a school psychologist's evaluation. They determine the student's cognitive capabilities, especially the possibility of any learning disability (which can then be further explored with the teachers

Table 6–1.   Working outline for SED case evaluation

Outline element	Sources of information			
	Referral information	Team meeting	Child interview	Parent interview
Presenting problems				
Past problems				
Interventions				
Review for other diagnoses				
Personal history				
Medical				
Developmental				
Social				
Family history				
Parents				
Stressors				
Test results				

Note.   SED = seriously emotionally disturbed.

and the parents for their observations). Frequently a school psychologist will perform more definitive tests when a learning disability is suspected after the basic screening. When past achievement test results are included, the student's rate of progress can also be ascertained.

Finally, the school psychologist's interpretation of the case is an important stepping-stone for the consultant. The school psychologist's opinion may be confirmed by the psychiatric consultation, or it may suggest diagnostic possibilities that must be clarified and issues that need further exploration with school staff and family.

2. Previous Evaluations

Formal reports of previous school (or community) evaluations can be very important to appreciate the ongoing history of a pupil's problems in school. For secondary school students, such reports often contain the only information available concerning past educational history, as current staff may have little knowledge about an adolescent's grade school performance. These reports also allow a consultant to review the past history of a case more economically and efficiently. They are preferable to extensive written anecdotal material, which is common in student files but generally too time consuming to wade through.

If such reports don't exist, it can be very difficult to learn an older pupil's past school history. However, a student's transcript may provide a good summary of academic performance, absences, conduct and socialization marks, and teachers' comments. Also, the summary report of group intelligence and achievement tests obtained at regular intervals by schools can indicate academic progress.

3. Teacher Behavior Checklist

The time available for the consultant to interview the current teacher(s) is limited. Therefore, the more the psychiatrist or psychologist appreciates the teacher's present concerns about a pupil before the team meeting, the better he or she can explore and clarify the teacher's observations during the initial team meeting, rather than risk achieving only a superficial understanding.

The Teacher's Report Form (TRF) developed by Achenbach (1991b) is suggested as a prototype checklist to be completed by the referring teacher. The initial part of this instrument allows the teacher to globally rate the student's academic and socialization skills. Space is allotted for the teacher to anecdotally summarize his or her concerns about the child.

The second section of the TRF allows the teacher to rate behavioral and mood items according to a three-point frequency/severity scale. This part allows the consultant to survey the teacher's main concerns (and to later be sure that all of these major items have been reviewed with the teacher). The accompanying profile of T scores for the narrow-band scales provides an additional overview of the type and severity of a student's school problems according to the teacher, and can provide valuable, objective supplemental information.

Use of such a standardized form offers several advantages. It allows teachers to economically summarize how they observe a student, rather than just spend time in anecdotal description. Teachers generally appreciate such organized forms amidst all their required paperwork. Use of a common instrument is especially helpful when the observations of several teachers are being compared (e.g., for secondary school students). Also, if the same checklist was used in the past, the past and present checklists can easily be compared to assess progress or deterioration; the same holds true for future assessments of outcome.

4. Parent Behavior Checklist

The reasons for obtaining a behavior checklist from the parent— for example, the TRF's companion Child Behavior Checklist (Achenbach 1991a)—parallel the reasons for obtaining a teacher checklist. Given the time constraints of a consultation but the need for thoroughness, the consultant needs a head start in appreciating the parent's concerns, which the information of a checklist can provide. The comparison of both teacher and parent checklists before the team meeting also allows the psychiatrist to question the teacher about symptoms that concern the parent but that the teacher may not have noted.

During the interview of the parent, the psychiatrist or psychologist can double-check the items checked as "very true or often true" on the parent checklist to be sure that all of the parent's primary concerns have been explored, because sometimes such concerns will not be mentioned spontaneously by the parent. A parent may initially be reluctant to admit to any problems with the child at home, but gentle confrontation with their checklist ratings can encourage disclosure. It is always desirable to obtain checklists from both parents; contrasting ratings can be very revealing.

Finally, use of parent checklists serves a remaining basic function: encouragement of collaboration between school staff and family, which is a necessity in the treatment of SED students. Collection of the checklist by the staff emphasizes their need to more fully understand the pupil's functioning at home to enable comprehensive treatment planning. Conversely, completion of the checklist 1) can signal to the parent that the school recognizes the need to work with parents and 2) can serve as an initial indication to the parent that he or she needs to work with school staff for the good of the student. Thus, mutual engagement is promoted, and the chances of a counterproductive adversarial relationship are diminished.

C. INITIAL MEETING WITH MULTIDISCIPLINARY TEAM

Review of the previously described preevaluation material helps to prepare the consultant to use the initial meeting with the educational staff more efficiently. Educators are appreciative when the consultant demonstrates that he or she has reviewed the material, which will enhance both the collaborative effort and the efficiency of the meeting. Time is limited for all parties, and staff can get frustrated if they have to cover the referral material again for an unprepared consultant.

The meeting with the educational staff occurs just before the student and the parent(s) are interviewed. The usual participants are the school psychologist who evaluated the child and key staff from the child's school such as the teacher(s), guidance counselor, and principal (or assistant principal). If a community therapist is involved, his or her participation should be encouraged, although it may be difficult to arrange. First, each educator should be encouraged to briefly present his or her observations and concerns about the student. In each instance the consultant should ask questions to clarify and expand, much as he or she would do when taking a history of present illness from parents. Notes from the review of the referral material should then be reexamined to ensure that those issues, as well as the teacher checklist items that were rated the most serious, have been addressed.

Finally, the team members' knowledge of the child's history outside of the school environment should be briefly surveyed (using the working outline's categories). Although school staff's information in these areas is often incomplete and anecdotal, their responses may suggest further important questions to be reviewed with the child and the parent(s). For example, a teacher may reveal that the child is suspected of running the streets while the parent is at bars, information a parent wouldn't spontaneously disclose. The consultant should emerge from the team meeting with a good understanding of the staff's view of the child and the family. Although the ensuing interviews with the child and family should be comprehensive, the educators' information will influence what areas are stressed and probed.

D. STUDENT INTERVIEW

This consultation is a "big deal" to any student because so many "important" people are involved and because the student knows it may change his or her life in school. Thus, interviewing the student first may diffuse understandable nervousness in younger students and may result in the appreciation and cooperation of the older student who wants his or her side of the story heard first.

A condensed working outline for the suggested interview with any student of kindergarten age or older is presented in Table 6–2. This interview parallels other established semistructured mental state exams, while being more "student friendly" (i.e., addressing more school issues). It is designed as a comprehensive series of probes that each can be expanded as necessary. Open-ended questions to encourage content should be combined with the inquiries about specific symptoms. The interview begins with the student discussing easy but important areas and moves to more intensive questions about possible specific symptoms.

The student should first be asked if he or she understands why he or she is being interviewed today, and if there are any questions about this interview. If the student does not understand the purpose of the consultation, then the psychiatrist or psychologist should explain that the school staff have concerns about his or her problems in school that they have just discussed with the consultant. Now the psychiatrist or psychologist wants to understand the student's side of the story, as well as explore other potential problem areas. The information won't be told to the parents (except if danger is involved), but it will be discussed with the school staff so they can better understand how to help the pupil. After this explanation, the student should again be asked for any questions.

Next, the student should be asked to describe any problems or worries that he or she may have about anything—school, friends, or home. Any response should be adequately expanded. Many children

Table 6–2.   Student interview for SED case evaluation

Introduction	Mood
Current (and past) problems	General
24-hour day	Anger
School (subjects, teachers, peers)	Fear
After school (friends and activities)	Sadness
Home (parents, stressors)	Mini neuroeducational exam
Medical complaints and sleep	Conclusion

are very open at this point, whereas others say little (and should not be pressed because information often flows later in the interview once they are more relaxed and trusting).

A helpful next step is to review the student's "24-hour day," both to get necessary information and to relax the student and encourage him or her to believe that you are trustworthy and sincerely interested in what he or she has to say. The flow of questions moves from school to play activities with friends (for secondary students, include substance use and exposure to substance use) to home life (including disciplinary practices, abuse, and other stressor experiences). In general, the consultant is interested in what the student says spontaneously about each part of the day, as well as determining the student's positive and negative observations and acquiring more standard specific information.

Specific inquiry about school can begin with what the student likes and dislikes about school currently, as well as whether the student even wants to attend school. Memories of past school experiences should be encouraged, and these memories should be compared with the present setting. Any academic difficulty admitted to by the pupil should be assessed by helping the student describe or pinpoint in his or her own words exactly how he or she experiences the problem (helpful information for diagnosis of a learning disability). Attitude toward the teacher(s) can then be discussed, as well as what makes the teacher yell at the student. Peer interaction should be surveyed (e.g., specific friends and enemies, recess activities, and how the student thinks other students regard him or her). The child should be asked how the parent(s) are reacting to his or her school difficulties. Finally, the student's true awareness of the problems and his or her self-developed solutions should be reviewed.

After the inquiry about the 24-hour day, the student should be ready for more typical "psychiatric" questions, especially about mood. The consultant can begin with inquiries about physical complaints and sleep habits. When inquiring about nighttime experiences, it is logical to ask about psychotic symptoms (e.g., shadows or sounds or unusual experiences that also occur during the day). Then the student can be asked about his or her usual mood (and most common second-place mood). The consultant is then interested in how the pupil experiences the major mood states of happiness, sadness, anger, and fear. Each of these mood states should be surveyed for associated specific psychopathology.

A brief developmental examination (e.g., of coordination) of the consultant's choosing can then be conducted, and the student can demonstrate what he or she is currently doing in reading, arithmetic, and spelling classes (to further observe for any possible learning disability). This section of the interview can be undertaken earlier to relax students who are reluctant to talk or to provide a rest from just talking for younger students.

In conclusion, the child can be asked again whether he or she has any remaining questions. Or there may be something that the doctor forgot to ask that would be important to know about.

E. PARENT INTERVIEW

While the parent(s) of the student is waiting during the child's interview, a staff member (ideally the school psychologist or an SED social worker, if present) can make valuable use of the time to interview the parent. Reasons for today's consultation, as well as the actual process itself, can again be explained and clarified, which may save the consultant time and diffuse anxiety or anger based on misunderstanding. The parent may have questions about the child's schooling or testing that can be reviewed. Also, extra information can be gathered to supplement the consultant's history. In particular, the staff member can ask about other services the child and family are currently receiving and how the delivery of that intervention is progressing (looking particularly for practical roadblocks that must be overcome to adequately secure consistent delivery). The same questions can be asked about past services.

An abbreviated working outline for the suggested parent interview is presented in Table 6–3. Much like the interview of the student, this semistructured interview of the parent(s) is meant to emphasize school issues, past and present. When the consultant begins to interview the parent(s), much the same opening that was used with the

child can be repeated. The discussion of confidentiality should indicate that relevant history will be shared with the team and a confidential report will be prepared (the family should already have signed an
appropriate release for the school).

The interview can then progress to any concerns the parent has
about the child in or out of school, first in the present and then in the
past. Each worry must be fully developed by the consultant because
each worry usually suggests the possibility of a psychiatric disorder
that must be clarified through specific questioning. Probes should
then be done to complete the comprehensive survey for major diagnoses. A final review of the parent behavior checklist can be useful to
ensure that the consultant does not overlook any serious symptom
that the parent has forgotten to mention at the time of the interview.
Finally, it should be stressed that the parent's information about the
child's past school functioning is very important, especially with older
students for whom staffs often have limited information about grade
school functioning.

The next section of the parent interview can focus on the child's
personal history: problems during pregnancy and delivery, medical
history, language and motor development, and socialization skills
(peer relationships and activities and substance use history in older
students). If previous psychological intervention has not already been
covered adequately, this is an appropriate time to do so.

The last section of the parent interview focuses on parent educational and psychiatric history, marital status, and student experience
of abuse and other stressors. Parenting practices can be surveyed, es-

Table 6–3.   Parent interview for SED case evaluation

Introduction	Family history
Current problems	Parents (medical, educational,
Past problems (and treatment)	and psychiatric)
Review of major DSM-III-R diagnoses	Marriage
Personal history	Parenting practices
Medical	Stresses (abuse)
Developmental	Extended family (genetics)
Social	Conclusion

pecially how parents handle the child's problems at home. The parent's explanation of the child's problems at school and home should be ascertained, as well as how the parent deals with those difficulties.

Finally, the interview can end as the child interview does, with the consultant inquiring whether there are any additional questions or any integral history that was not brought up. The parent(s) will usually want some feedback at this point. They can be assured that information will be provided after the next step: discussion with the team members.

F. FEEDBACK TO TEAM AND COLLABORATIVE TREATMENT PLANNING

Feedback to the educational team members has several purposes. It summarizes the consultant's comprehensive view of the child and the family, as well as providing a diagnostic formulation for consideration by the whole team. Such information increases the team's understanding of the child, filling in new facts and often correcting former misconceptions. Frequently some of the staff may be quite upset with the student or the family, or both, and such a comprehensive overview can rekindle necessary empathy. Finally, this process has an inherent teaching function for the staff (e.g., suggesting further questions they could have asked or other hypotheses that could have been considered). This educational aspect can prove valuable in their future work with problematic students.

First, the interview with the child should be summarized, highlighting both positive and negative aspects. Special attention should be addressed to comparing the consultant's findings with those of the other team members. Staff are very interested in issues that they considered but couldn't fully explore with the child. Next, the interview with the parent(s) should be summarized in a similar manner, addressing key points of the history. Special attention should be directed to confirming or correcting information that staff disclosed during the initial meeting of the team.

After the diagnostic formulation (DSM-III-R diagnoses [American Psychiatric Association 1987]) has been presented, discussion among all the team members can then progress. This interaction is quite dependent on the quality and relevance of the consultant's feedback (i.e., how directly the overview addressed the hypotheses and observations of the other team members). Give and take should be stimulated by the consultant to ensure that the diagnostic formulation is agreed on by the team as a sound basis for treatment planning.

Next, the intervention designed by the team should focus not only on school intervention, but also on what community resources are needed by the child and the family. Thus, the previous feedback to the team takes on added importance; the more everyone understands the total picture, the more they can appreciate what treatment should follow. This understanding allows frank discussion of what can actually be arranged or what priorities are most crucial. A particular intervention may not seem possible until one team member suggests a creative solution.

The consultant can initiate discussion of school intervention by suggesting specific targets and treatment approaches. The school staff can then help expand these ideas—in particular, the actual delivery of the specific interventions. The crux of the matter is the translation of treatment ideas into actions that can be adequately and consistently accomplished in the school environment. Subsequent discussion among the team must be frank in regard to the staff's intervention capabilities, their ability to consistently provide the necessary treatment, and the availability of ongoing treatment consultation within the school system. A school staff member must be assigned to be responsible for coordinating the intervention plan in the school.

Treatment planning should be completed by determining the non-educational needs of the student and family, which must be addressed using community psychological resources. Staff should then focus on arranging to provide for such needs. Some families will need only a list of resources and will then follow through, whereas others will require a staff member to help them procure the proper resources or arrange for agency involvement. At this point, the consultant may be called on to take one or more of several possible steps: arranging hospitalization, contacting the family physician to request a medication trial or adjustment, updating the child's current therapist about the consultation and team findings, or procuring a specialized referral.

G. FEEDBACK TO PARENT(S) AND STUDENT

Feedback to the family that reviews the findings of the consultation and the team discussion should be given by the child mental health professional and the educator who will continue to be most integrally involved with the child and family. Giving feedback with large numbers of team members should be avoided to prevent intimidation and to ensure that the family hears the communication of one or two voices clearly. Initially, it is preferable to give feedback to the parent(s) alone to promote an atmosphere for frank discussion. However, at times adolescents should also be involved (e.g., when it is important that all family members hear exactly the same feedback).

First, the diagnostic formulation should be explained to the parent(s) in understandable terms, including reasoning based on the background history. The parents usually appreciate a brief education about the diagnosis(diagnoses), along with any prognostic statements that are possible. Questions should always be encouraged. Next, the consultant should explain how the treatment plan will be implemented both in and out of school. This part of the feedback to the parents is probably the most vital. If successful, it can help establish healthy cooperation with school staff and ensure that the family will truly move to obtain the community resources that are suggested. Finally, the consultant should summarize the feedback and conclude by ensuring that everyone understands their responsibility in the execution of the treatment plan.

Feedback should then be given to the student, duplicating but simplifying what was said to the parent. The pupil should be told what the problems are, why they are probably occurring, and what everyone can do to help, both in and out of school. Questions can then be encouraged. If the student's response is minimal, he or she should be encouraged to explain back what was just said, to attempt to ensure some understanding and to further stimulate questions now rather than later in the car as the family returns home.

The question of self-referral may arise. If parents ask for an appointment with the consultant, the consultant can indicate appreciation. It may be wisest to offer a few other resources and encourage parents to check with their child's pediatrician, relatives, or friends before they decide to begin sending their child for therapy with the consultant. The consulting child psychologist or psychiatrist should reassure the family of his or her willingness to share the results of the consultation with whomever they choose once they give permission.

H. REPORT PREPARATION

The child psychiatrist's or psychologist's report on the SED consultation should never be taken for granted as just another report. Generally, it serves as the most comprehensive report of the student's problems in an SED child's school file. This write-up should summarize the student's present and past history in school and at home, state the diagnostic rationale, and outline the total treatment plan, highlighting especially specific thinking for school intervention. School staff, present and future, will value this report highly if it is properly accomplished. It can become the keystone of the student's educational future, not only ensuring basic understanding among school staff who will be working with the student, but also fostering empathy.

The report can follow the working outline of Table 6–1, with the addition of the diagnostic formulation and discussion and the comprehensive treatment plan for the child both in and out of school. Specific school interventions should be recommended for staff to develop. Community interventions can only be suggested, as they should be the parent's responsibility to arrange. Overall, the report should be thorough but not exhaustive. If the report is not "user friendly," staff will find it overwhelming, confusing, or impractical and useless, and the potential value of the consultation can easily be lost. An example of a model case report is provided in Appendix 6–1. The subject of this report is a grade-school boy who was judged in need of SED programming.

I. SUMMARY

This chapter presents a model for an SED case evaluation, a consultation that child mental health professionals commonly perform but that has few standard guidelines in any literature. The model emphasizes review of proper referral material to enhance efficient use of the actual consultation time, close collaboration with educational personnel at every step, thoroughness of both the school and the home history, comprehensive and practical treatment planning, and understandable feedback to the staff, the student, and the parents to better ensure actualization of the suggested interventions. Except for the extra focus on school, the model is based on standard evaluation procedures.

Although SED case evaluation may be considered a specialized case consultation, the same principles apply to any case evaluation of a child referred by a school, whether the evaluation is done in the private office of a child mental health professional or during contracted consultation time. Although the proposed model may have to be condensed or adapted, certain guidelines remain important: thoroughness, collaboration, and coherent explanations and practical recommendations.

J. REFERENCES

Achenbach TM: Manual for the Child Behavior Checklist/4-18 and Profile. Burlington, VT, Department of Psychiatry, University of Vermont, 1991a

Achenbach TM: Manual for the Teacher's Report Form and Profile. Burlington, VT, Department of Psychiatry, University of Vermont, 1991b

American Psychiatric Association: Diagnostic and Statistical Manual of Mental Disorders, 3rd Edition, Revised. Washington, DC, American Psychiatric Association, 1987

Berkovitz IH, Seliger JS (eds): Expanding Mental Health Interventions in Schools, Vol 1. Dubuque, IA, Kendall/Hunt, 1985

Berkowitz MI: A Primer on School Mental Health Consultation. Springfield, IL, Charles C Thomas, 1975

Jellinek MS: School consultation: evolving issues. J Am Acad Child Adolesc Psychiatry 29:311–314, 1990

Appendix 6–1.   Sample Consultation Report

SCHOOL CONSULTATION CENTER

Student: Date of Consultation:

DOB: Location:

                                                      Consultant:

IDENTIFYING INFORMATION:

Peter is a 9-year-old Caucasian boy who currently lives with his mother.
He attends third grade with resource room help for a learning disability.
He was referred by the school for diagnostic evaluation and treatment recommendations concerning his increasing difficulties in the classroom. The
history was provided by school personnel and the mother.

PRESENTING HISTORY:

Peter is a young boy who has been having academic and behavioral difficulties since the beginning of his schooling. He had to repeat second
grade. He was referred for evaluation this year due to increasing concerns
about his behavior and mood.

School personnel present as their primary concern Peter's level of depression. He is seen as sad and gradually withdrawing more and more from
peer interaction. He is described as isolated and has no good friends. He
frequently downs himself, saying that he is "no good" and "ugly," and he is
preoccupied with morbid themes. Six months ago, he wrote a note in
school which said, "This is my chance to kill myself. I love you, mom." He
also wrote a note saying, "If there were no TV, I would slap myself around.
If there was no TV, I would commit murder." He has made no suicide attempts of which the school is aware.

As for other school concerns, over the past few months staff has also become concerned about his level of aggression. He was involved in frequent
fights, kicking and choking other students. Also, his attention span is limited, and he is distractible and impulsive in the classroom. Peter had been
on methylphenidate several years ago, which teachers felt improved his attention span and decreased his hyperactivity. The mother reportedly discontinued the medication because she was concerned about side effects. In
addition, Peter on one occasion told a teacher that he heard a voice calling
his name. There have been no other reported hallucinations. His thoughts

have always been clear and coherent, and no other strange behaviors have been noted. Staff are not sure about a learning disability, given his poor concentration. Testing has revealed an average IQ with variable achievement test results.

The mother is aware of the school's concerns but reports that she is less concerned about his behavior at home. In fact, she reported feeling "railroaded" by the school into the evaluation. She has noticed Peter to be depressed in the past but feels that he is doing much better over the past 6 months. She does note that he has a poor self-image and tends to put himself down. She said he often appears sad to other people but feels that this is because he is similar to her and neither one of them shows a great deal of emotion. She notes no sleep disturbance. His appetite is described as variable, but there has been no significant weight change over the last several months. The mother reported that he is quite slow moving and very quiet in the morning but seems to get "hyped up" by mid-morning. She has noted no suicidal ideation at home but recalls that he witnessed a local official's suicide on television and shortly thereafter an adult friend of hers committed suicide. This man was the husband of one of Peter's babysitters. He seemed to talk a lot about this and seemed to read any newspaper article he found on suicide for a period of several months.

In regard to his hyperactivity, the mother states that since her son was very young "he has been like a greased pig." He is in constant motion. She still feels that she has to watch him closely in a shopping mall or he will run off. In a restaurant when he was younger, she described him as going into a "frenzy" and being uncontrollable. He has a limited attention span and is quite impulsive, risk-taking, and distractible.

In the review of other areas of symptomatology with her, when Peter is angry, he goes to his room and punches a pillow. The mother does not describe him as oppositional and is aware of no conduct problems such as stealing, destruction of public property, or cruelty to animals. She is aware of no drug or alcohol use. She does not see her son as an anxious child; he was fearful of the dark and water but is no longer. She describes no obsessions or compulsions and no anxieties associated with separation. The mother has never felt that Peter was grossly misinterpreting reality and has never thought that he was actively hallucinating or delusional.

In regard to his *personal history,* Peter was born approximately three weeks prior to term after the mother fell on ice and apparently ruptured her membranes. He was born via spontaneous vaginal delivery and had a birth weight of 7 lb. 101/2 oz. The mother recalls that he appeared somewhat blue at birth, but required no special resuscitation and went to a regular nursery. He sat at 6 months, walked at 1 year, and talked by 1 1/2 years.

The mother said he was always very active, even as an infant. She thinks he is smart enough to do his school work, although his performance has always been erratic. Concerning peers, the mother does not allow Peter to play with children in his neighborhood because she feels they are "bad kids" and will get him into trouble. Medically, he had a tonsillectomy at age 3 but no other surgeries. The mother reports that he has mild asthma and infrequently uses an inhaler. No other major medical problems were reported.

He saw a therapist 2 years ago for approximately 6 months on the advice of the school; she wasn't sure if it was helpful. She reported that currently Peter is in therapy again at the recommendation of the school. The mother reported that he had a trial of methylphenidate several years ago. She felt that it did slow him down but also made him appear "drugged out" and was concerned it was decreasing his appetite.

In regard to *family history,* the natural mother reported that she stopped school in the 11th grade (she now has her general equivalency diploma) and moved in with friends because her stepfather was verbally abusive. She described no learning disability or special-education services. When she was 15 years old, she reported that she accidentally took an overdose of Librium and spent a week in a general medical hospital. She has had no psychiatric care and minimized any current symptoms. Her older brother was a Vietnam veteran who abused alcohol and made a suicide attempt. Peter's natural father graduated from high school and has taken some college courses. He has no learning disabilities. He reportedly abused heroin in Vietnam and was an alcoholic. He was physically abusive to the mother but not to Peter. His problems led to divorce, and he now rarely sees Peter. The mother reports that financial concerns are the only current stress in the house.

MENTAL STATUS EXAMINATION:

Peter was a healthy-appearing boy who was alert and oriented and willingly entered the interview room. He had good hygiene and was dressed neatly and in an age-appropriate manner. His speech was soft but clear, coherent, and goal-directed, and his use and comprehension of language were age-appropriate. His overall level of cognitive functioning was judged to be average. No unusual tics, tremors, or mannerisms were noted, and results of his neurological screening exam were within normal limits.

Most striking in this evaluation was the level of Peter's depression. His voice was soft and his affect was depressed. He smiled only twice, and then only briefly, during the entire evaluation. He described his mood as "bored" and felt like he really didn't enjoy anything. He described a decreased appetite. He felt his sleep was generally all right and described no diurnal variation in mood. He has thoughts of running away from home quite frequently although he said he would not because he has nowhere to go. He related that he has frequent thoughts of wishing he were dead. He discussed the suicide of his babysitter's husband. He stated that he has never considered killing himself and was confident that he never would. He stated that the "suicide note" from school was written out of anger and that he has never been actively suicidal.

Peter was fidgety with his hands during the evaluation but was basically still and attentive. However, he described himself in school as having difficulty paying attention, finding it difficult to sit in his seat, and impulsively calling out. He recalled that the methylphenidate seemed to slow him down but he felt it made him "abnormal" and "too slowed down" so he couldn't run around and enjoy himself.

When he gets angry, Peter says he feels like punching people but he tries hard to resist this. He denied frequent fighting, stealing, destruction of public property, or involvement with the police. He denied any drug or alcohol use. He gave no history of anxiety. His thoughts were clear and logical, and he denied any hallucinations or delusions.

In regard to important areas in a young boy's life, Peter said that school was "okay." He felt that he had a lot of problems with mathematics and enjoyed reading more. He said that his classmates don't like him and often tease him. He described going up to a group of peers on the playground and having them all moved away, saying that they didn't want to be his friend. After school, he goes to a special program in the school for children with working parents. He said he mostly just runs around during this time but seemed to enjoy it.

At home, he said, "All I do is just go and sit." He described sitting on the couch with his mother all evening watching television. He has no peer interaction after school. He said sometimes his mother gets quite angry at him and says that she wishes that he wasn't her son. Occasionally, she will get angry and throw a shoe at him, but nothing more physical. He and his mother can also have good times, and he enjoys talking and walking with her. He said little about his father but allowed that he would like to see him.

DISCUSSION:

From the history and current mental status examination, it appears that Peter has dysthymia (chronic depression). He has a long-standing depressive syndrome including sad mood and affect, anhedonia, feelings of inadequacy, and some disturbance in appetite. This disorder is currently causing the most problems for Peter and is thus the primary diagnosis. Furthermore, these symptoms may be of sufficient severity to fulfill diagnostic criteria for a major depression, a possibility that must be discussed with his current therapist.

In addition to the above-noted depressive features, Peter has a long-standing history consistent with attention-deficit hyperactivity disorder (ADHD); he is hyperactive, impulsive, distractible, and has a limited attention span. It appears as though he had a positive response to methylphenidate in the past but may have had some side effects that could have been better managed. It is important to treat this illness concurrently with his dysthymia as it is likely an exacerbating factor in his depression.

EDUCATIONAL RECOMMENDATIONS:

Peter will require an SED classroom to adequately address his serious and multiple classroom needs: academic, social, and emotional. Any learning disability should be better defined and specifically addressed. Self-management techniques for his ADHD symptoms may prove helpful, as well as the behavioral structure of an SED classroom. Social skills can be better assessed and taught. His depressive symptoms can be addressed in several ways: positive feedback, warm staff interaction, arrangement of situations for success, and affective training. Staff should work closely with his therapist, and especially report deterioration and suicidal symptoms.

OTHER NONEDUCATIONAL SUGGESTIONS:

1. Given the combination of depressive and attentional symptoms and the fact that his trial of methylphenidate was complicated by troublesome side effects, it is suggested that Peter have a trial of desipramine. The mother was quite open to this suggestion and gave her permission for us to talk to the therapist to determine how this might be arranged, especially if the therapist's observation also pointed toward major depression.

2. It is also suggested that Peter should continue in individual therapy. Again, the mother gave her permission for us to contact the therapist concerning this evaluation and its suggestions. The therapist must especially continue to monitor for worsening depression; if Peter becomes more depressed and suicidal, hospitalization should be considered.

3. Finally, there is concern about the mother's own psychological needs, which will also be reviewed with the therapist to ascertain what he is doing or could arrange in this regard.

CHAPTER SEVEN

Principles in Common School Case Consultations

Richard E. Mattison, M.D.

This chapter presents three common case consultations involving elementary, junior high, and high school students. In each case, the consultant plays a different essential role, although treatment is the main issue. First, the case is described, including the consultation process itself. Then, the important consultation issues are discussed as they arose during the flow of the case. Finally, the principles common to all three cases are summarized at the end of the chapter. Common consultation needs of school systems are presented in the next chapter.

The primary focus of each case presentation is consultant interaction with school staff. Thus, the treatment discussion will concentrate more on the school environment than on the separate intervention needs of the child and family. Furthermore, an attempt has been made to select mainly references from school literature for educators. Research studies pertaining to the school functioning of students with psychiatric disorders are not plentiful in any literature, but reports are emerging that can be recommended. Thus, consultants can recommend these books and articles knowing that they are more likely to be available to and read by school personnel.

A. ELEMENTARY SCHOOL (CASE 1)

The following case example illustrates the multifaceted process of a private clinician developing a school intervention plan for a boy with attention-deficit hyperactivity disorder (ADHD) with the school staff who referred the boy.

Alan, an 8-year-old black boy in second grade, was referred for the first time to a child psychiatrist in a local community mental health clinic because the school staff told the mother they were worried about hyperactivity, as well as the boy's low self-esteem, poor academic performance, increasing defiance, and disruptive peer interaction. The mother understood the school's concerns and was aware that her son was not doing as well as he did in first grade. He complained that the teacher and peers picked on him. His grades were not as good as in the past, and at times he came home discouraged about his day at school, or at other times even wished he could stay home and not go to school. Past teachers had expressed some concerns similar to those of the current staff, but they thought he would grow out of his problems.

The mother gave a history consistent with ADHD. She had been able to tolerate the symptomatology in the past, but it was starting to become more bothersome to her. She still felt much warmth for her son and did not regard him as a bad boy. She generally felt that she could control him, but he was becoming verbally defiant and she more often had to repeat herself to get him to do things. They lived in a poor neighborhood, and she did not like the kids on the streets. Her son was getting into fights, and she was limiting him more to the house so he wouldn't get into trouble. However, then he would get irritable because there wasn't much for him to do in the house. His mood was often still good, but she could see him looking sad more often (e.g., after school or when things didn't go well outside).

The mother and the boy's father had never married and only lived together until the boy was about 1 year old. By the mother's report, the father drank too much and had a bad temper. Indeed, those problems ended the relationship, especially when he began to push the mother around and scream intolerantly at the baby. According to the father's own mother, Alan's problems reminded her much of when the father was a boy. The mother had moved back in with her parents; she and the boy lived downstairs and her parents upstairs in a two-flat tenement. The grandparents could tolerate just so much of his exuberance and now were tending to yell at him more frequently, which only further distressed the boy and made him irritable or sad. The mother was working long hours during the day and coming home very tired; she also felt guilty because she thought that she should go back to school and better herself. She was increasingly upset that she was always grumpy with Alan, and less frequently felt up to playing with him. She had no medical or psychiatric history, although she was feeling increasingly frustrated and sad with the course of their lives.

Alan's mental state was consistent with his mother's observations. Although he was fidgety and talkative, he was open and cooperative. His mood was good except for sadness and irritability during discussion of school. He was getting into trouble for talking and not getting his work done, and he didn't like it when his teacher scolded him or the kids teased him about his troubles. He was starting to get into fights. None of the work was too hard. School wasn't as much fun as last year, but he still liked it. His mother got angry at him sometimes about school. She also was more irritable at home, and they were doing fewer fun things together. He was getting bored staying inside so much, although he understood that many kids in the neighborhood were troublemakers.

A teacher's checklist (the Teacher's Report Form; Achenbach 1991b) had been completed and was striking for ADHD symptoms, indeed, at a more severe level than the mother's checklist (the Child Behavior Checklist; Achenbach 1991a) had indicated. Furthermore, the teacher also appeared quite concerned that the boy's verbal (and now physical) aggression and temper tantrums were disrupting his peer relationships, and that his moodiness with crying and noncompliance was affecting his already compromised work performance. No psychoeducational testing had been done.

Given the worrisome nature of the teacher's checklist, the psychiatrist phoned her and confirmed that she was indeed worried. Therefore, with the mother's approval, a conference was arranged after school one day to include the teacher, the principal, the guidance counselor, and the school district's psychologist if he could attend. The end of the school day worked out well for all the staff, as everyone was able to attend without interruptions. The child psychiatrist opened by thanking the staff for the referral and noting that the mother was quite supportive of the meeting. He suggested that a good place to begin was the staff's concerns about the boy.

The primary teacher described Alan as a boy with moderate ADHD symptomatology. She did not suspect any learning disorder, but thought rather that his poor concentration and easy distractibility were interfering with his academic progress. She was aware of the poor area where he lived as well as the mother's struggles, but felt that his symptoms were not just a reaction to those stresses. In contrast to the degree of her concerns expressed in the checklist and over the phone, she was pleased with the boy's social skills. She did not feel that he was too aggressive, but rather that when he was in a bad mood he was more quick to yell or swing at peers . Though generally happy, he was often moody when school wasn't going well. She was most worried that Alan's problems were getting worse, and she didn't want to see that happen as she liked the boy.

The teacher went on to note that she may have overemphasized his problems to the psychiatrist because she had two other hyperactive boys in her class who were much worse than Alan; thus, perhaps she was overreacting out of frustration over this especially stressful year. She felt she was good with hyperactive children and did not shy away from having them in her class. However, this year's class was more overwhelming than usual, and she needed more help.

The psychiatrist asked what the staff knew about the mother. They liked her but noted her decreasing availability during the year and that she also looked more harried. Alan complained to them about being kept inside or grounded too much. They felt that the mother was partly being protective as he would be especially vulnerable in their tough neighborhood. The guidance counselor and principal knew Alan casually and liked him, but their primary knowledge was through their school team that monitored children with problems. The school psychologist had not met him.

At this point, based on his interviews with Alan and his mother and on the information gained from the meeting with the school staff, the psychiatrist began to explain that his working diagnosis was ADHD with reactive mood symptoms (the presumptive diagnosis and treatment plan had already been discussed with the mother). He, too, doubted any learning disability, although that question should be re-evaluated after seeing the response to the proposed interventions. He thought a methylphenidate (Ritalin) trial was indicated. The mother and boy should be educated about ADHD, and their other needs would gradually be clarified (e.g., further assessment of the mother's mental state and her needs for support). With school staff present, planning for appropriate school intervention could begin, and sugges-tions could be generated for after-school activities to help Alan and his mother with that growing problem.

The staff concurred with the diagnosis and treatment plan. The teacher and the counselor said that they had been leery of methylphe-nidate in the past, but over time they had come to believe that it was beneficial to many hyperactive children. Their main concern now was properly communicating their observations about the medication's ef-fects on the child to the doctor. Too often, they said, doctors had little or no contact with school staff. The psychiatrist explained his check-list monitoring procedure as well as his use of periodic phone con-tacts, and the staff were reassured.

Next, school issues were addressed, first by assessing the staff's knowledge about ADHD. The expertise of the primary teacher in deal-ing with hyperactive children proved to be rather limited (i.e., based more on experience than on training). For example, she placed such children by her desk to help them focus on their work. She also looked out for them on the playground so that they wouldn't get into trouble. Because they often got yelled at by others, she went out of her way to praise them for positive accomplishments. Despite these helpful inter-ventions, she felt that she ought to understand them better and know more intervention steps. The guidance counselor and the principal felt much like the teacher: their knowledge about ADHD was rudimentary and they needed more education. In contrast, the school psychologist had more understanding and was aware of behavioral intervention techniques, but had little time to help teachers apply such methods.

To address the ADHD education needs of the school's staff, the psychiatrist offered to begin by providing a general lecture-and-answer presentation; the staff determined that there was time during an upcoming in-service day. In addition, the psychologist offered to discuss on that same day specific behavioral interventions that regular-education teachers could use with ADHD children in their classrooms. A separate time was also set for the teacher, school psychologist, and psychiatrist to meet and design a classroom behavioral intervention plan for Alan. The psychologist agreed to meet every 2 weeks with the teacher to monitor the plan. The psychiatrist proposed that the teacher become the "local expert" to assist other teachers in the school with future ADHD children; the teacher appeared open to this idea.

The discussion next moved to improving activities for the boy after school. Alan was faced with provocation in a tough, poor neighborhood or boredom at home with an irritable mother. The psychiatrist asked the staff about community opportunities available for their students, both after school and on weekends. One staff member noted that there was an after-school program where kids played under supervision and also were assisted with homework until their parents picked them up. Children wishing to get involved in sports were taken to their practices and games if necessary. That program might be especially good for Alan because it also featured positive male role models to help minority boys deal with the many neighborhood problems that they face, such as violence and drugs. Another staff member thought that two local churches offered Saturday functions as well as summer programs. The guidance counselor volunteered to track down those resources and then offer them to the mother, as well as to explore her idea of a Big Brother program. Thus, the boy would benefit in many ways, and the mother would gain some relief and a little more time for herself.

As for the other two problem boys in the teacher's classroom, the counselor noted that she was meeting with one boy's parents to encourage them to seek help from community resources. The principal said that in the past he had successfully dealt with the same parents concerning another sibling, and he volunteered to sit in with the counselor to use his influence. Finally, the staff noted that the school team had decided to refer the second problem boy to the school psychologist for further evaluation, which hopefully would then lead to proper intervention.

Thus, the meeting ended in a satisfactory matter. The teacher was pleased, but she knowingly observed that the real work had just begun.

Discussion:

1. This typical elementary school case illustrates several issues that are important to clinicians working with school staffs concerning a child with ADHD. First, ascertainment of the child's functioning at school was an important part of the initial evaluation to confirm the diagnosis and shape the clinician's thinking as he or she formulates a comprehensive treatment plan. This integral step was accomplished by obtaining the parent's history concerning school and doing preliminary screening with the Teacher Behavior Checklist, followed by a subsequent phone call to the child's teacher. In this manner, the child psychiatrist or psychologist can efficiently and economically determine what the appropriate next step should be to address the child's needs in school. Furthermore, these early contacts are appreciated by teachers and prepare the way for an optimal working relationship with school personnel. Finally, school input was especially vital in this case of a disadvantaged minority boy in whom potential ADHD symptoms had to be differentiated from a reaction to environmental stresses.

2. Basic understanding of the school environment was required to successfully initiate work with the school staff. Parental approval was required for the psychiatrist to contact or meet with school personnel; thus, the mother had completed the psychiatrist's standard consent form. The meeting was arranged with all school staff involved with the boy at a convenient time. Such times usually are soon after end-of-the-day dismissal, before school begins, or during set meeting times for teams that monitor problem children. The meeting concerning Alan demonstrates how essential it is to have all school staff present. If all staff had not been present, his treatment plan probably would not have evolved so smoothly, nor would everyone have had the same important initial understanding of the case and the overall treatment approach.

3. An actual meeting with school personnel is indispensable to supplement any office evaluation when it is determined that the child is showing significant problems in school. Without such a meeting in the above case, the child psychiatrist would not have understood that the primary teacher was actually optimistic about Alan rather than pessimistic, and that other forces were affecting her interaction with the boy (i.e., two other boys who had even more serious classroom problems than Alan had and little immediate help on the horizon). Furthermore, the availability of a knowledgeable school psychologist would have gone unrecognized, and as a result, a valuable resource would not have been used. Such meetings also help the clinician learn more about his or her first impression of the parent(s) and family functioning. In addition, various staff were aware of possible community programs to mitigate the neighborhood problems and home boredom with which the boy and his mother were struggling. Such local knowledge is particularly helpful in inner-city neighborhoods, where a consultant may not be aware of crucial existent programs.

4. The working relationship with the school staff was further strengthened when the psychiatrist discussed his diagnostic reasoning and preliminary treatment planning and invited their reactions and questions. Staff input is important not only because it allows staff to make critical responses to the clinician's assessment, but also because this process aids the consultant in gauging the staff's empathy and understanding of the case, prerequisites for adequate care of the child in school. In the case of this school staff (without the school psychologist), their basic knowledge of ADHD probably would have been insufficient to care adequately for the child in school. A brief presentation about ADHD would have been appreciated, but it would have been insufficient to meet their true needs and thus would have had limited impact.

Also, in the case of ADHD children, staff may be so wary of methylphenidate because of negative media publicity that they undermine parental acceptance by painting a negative picture of this medication treatment. Such bias can also color their observations of the medication's true effects. In addition, some school personnel may have little tolerance for ADHD children and want them placed in another environment, even though they can commonly remain in a regular classroom if basic intervention is provided. Finally, many school staffs are unenthusiastic about working with outside professionals because they feel, too often correctly so, that their valuable school observations are neither sought nor listened to. Staff with such previous negative experience may unilaterally treat an ADHD child on their own, properly or improperly, believing that they have to do it by themselves without meaningful collaboration from community professionals.

5. School case consultations often evolve into system consultations. In particular, consultants are often faced with school staffs who must work with psychiatrically ill children but who have limited understanding of particular diagnoses or of the proper implementation of required treatment in the school. If the consultant faces this situation, he or she must first assess whether any current school staff person can fill an ongoing consultant role. Educators understandably learn better from fellow educators, a situation that holds true within any profession. Because the prevalence rate of ADHD is approximately 4%, school personnel must commonly deal with these children, many of whom can remain in regular classrooms with proper care. If the consultant does not find a base of sufficient working knowledge or a staff member for collaborative effort, then he or she should offer to help the school (or, ideally, the school district) develop its own resources for caring for ADHD children.

6. Staff cannot be adequately educated about ADHD (or any diagnosis) in one presentation, which too often is all they receive. Continuing education is required (e.g., provided by a staff person who takes an intensive summer course and then conveys that knowledge to his or her colleagues during the subsequent school year), supplemented by appropriate texts. Basic reading materials for educators are becoming more available, such as the following:

1. *Attention Deficit Hyperactivity Disorder: A Handbook for Diagnosis and Treatment* (Barkley 1990).
2. *Cognitive-Behavioral Therapy With ADHD: A Child, Family and School Model* (Braswell and Bloomquist 1991).

3. *Disruptive Behavior Disorders in Children: Treatment-Focused Assessment* (Breen and Altepeter 1990).

Also, recent issues of major educational journals have been devoted to ADHD: *School Psychology Review* (Volume 20, No. 2, 1991) and *Journal of Learning Disabilities* (Volume 24, No. 2–4, 1991).

Similarly, classroom intervention techniques cannot be acquired without ongoing instruction and experience. Generally, such ongoing coaching is best provided to teachers by a school psychologist. Teachers are familiar with behavioral modification, a key component in the care of ADHD children. The above books provide technical descriptions that teachers will find useful. A very practical manual also is published by Hawthorne Educational Services (1989): *The Attention Deficit Disorders Intervention Manual, School Version.*

Breen and Altepeter (1990) summarize principles that teachers must apply consistently to help ADHD children: positive individual relationships, clear communication, individualized teaching, firmness, proper seating, frequent rewards, work appropriate for the child's abilities, extra help, repeated directions, slowed pace, and appropriate energy outlets. Pfiffner and Barkley (1990) add the following: immediate deliverance of consequences, more powerful consequences, frequently rotated reinforcers, and anticipatory planning and prompting.

Cognitive self-management can also be used in the classroom (Zentall 1989). Such potential interventions are reviewed for educators by Hinshaw and Erhardt (1991) in a recent text on cognitive-behavioral therapy edited by Kendall (1991). These techniques include self-instruction and self-evaluation, anger management, and attribution training. However, the authors caution that these techniques have not yet proven to be as efficacious as expected. Further research is required, especially into the behavioral interventions that are necessary to enhance self-management approaches.

7. Finally, just as parents manage ADHD children better when their own needs are addressed, the same holds true for teachers. In the above case, the teacher was stressed by other more disruptive chil-

dren. The psychiatrist led the team toward resolution of those issues and consequently may have earned further gratitude from the
teacher. In turn, the teacher's thankfulness might then be trans-
lated into increased effort with the consultant's patient, as well as
more effort to better understand and properly care for ADHD children in her classroom and school. School consultants should appreciate the power they have to energize school staffs.

B. JUNIOR HIGH SCHOOL (CASE 2)

The following case example illustrates the collaboration between a
child psychologists and a school staff for the reintroduction of a
school-refusing teenage girl back into the classroom:

The parents of 13-year-old Betsy, a girl in seventh grade (her first
year of junior high school), brought her for private evaluation by a
child psychologist at the encouragement of her pediatrician. For the
past 6 weeks (since the Christmas holidays), she had missed school
because of abdominal pain. Extensive medical evaluation had revealed
no physical etiology. The parents were frustrated by the lack of diagnostic progress while still having to watch Betsy suffer. Two attempts
had been made to return her to school. During the first, she lasted only
a couple of hours before the school nurse called for the parents to pick
her up. During the second she could not even get out of the car because of the pain's intensity. The mother now stated that they were
waiting for a few days' freedom from pain before making another attempt; there had been some pain-free days, but not enough in a row.

A history revealed that Betsy had begun kindergarten with difficulty;
for the first month her mother had to taper her own presence there. The
current problem was the first major recurrence, though last year Betsy
had missed more days of school than usual. Betsy had never tolerated
being away from home well. She still liked having other girls spend the
night at her house, and last year she even had a problem going away for
a week with her grandparents during summer vacation.

Over the years, school had been marginally difficult for her. Betsy
had always required remedial reading and had never had many friends

except for one in the neighborhood. The parents had worried about how she would make the transition this year into a junior high school atmosphere, but they felt she had done better than expected. Currently, she did little during the day except for light homework, watching television, or playing in her room. She did not seem to enjoy family functions and even experienced some abdominal pain on those occasions. She seemed frustrated that she couldn't go back to school, but the parents were not struck by other evidence of depression or anxiety.

Family history revealed an older sister who had experienced similar difficulties for almost 3 years when she first began school, but who was now functioning well. The parents admitted to no past or current major stressors, except that their marriage had its ups and downs, although it was currently stable. The mother currently works, although she had taken off much time recently to help her daughter. Genetic history revealed only that the maternal grandmother had also experienced chronic abdominal pain that almost resulted in surgery last year; this grandmother frequently babysat for Betsy.

During her interview, Betsy showed little affect and no evidence of abdominal pain. Initially, she was mildly upset that there was so much emphasis on her returning to school, as if the doctors did not believe that she was really suffering pain. In summary, the pain was in her left lower quadrant and intermittent. Nothing seemed to make it worse or better, and there were no accompanying symptoms.

She vaguely recalled a similar problem when she was younger, but then nothing until last spring. Then she missed a few days of school at a time, and there were also some accompanying headaches. She didn't like the teacher she had because he was always yelling at the class (though not at her), and she had to work harder overall. She also had some worry about how she would cope in junior high.

From her point of view, the current year was proving difficult because of hard work and adjustment to all the new kids and teachers. She recalled missing a few days of school with headaches just after the Thanksgiving holiday and then missing the week before Christmas with the flu. Christmas vacation had gone well, but on the first day back to school the abdominal pain had occurred in the morning. It had not completely remitted since that time.

Overall, Betsy admitted to an "in-between" mood, which she thought was normal for her. She still preferred playing by herself or with her friend. She was not particularly depressed; she was more upset and angry that the pain was still occurring (as opposed to sad or worried about all the school she was missing). She admitted to an occasional verbal temper. As for anxiety, she was leery of scary movies, but her mother wouldn't allow her to watch them anyhow. She also didn't like being away from home. When asked what she would do if her class were to go on an appealing overnight field trip, Betsy first said her mother would chaperon. Asked what she would do if her mother couldn't go, she said she probably wouldn't go either. When asked if the trip was to Disney World, she said she might go then.

As for family life, Betsy vaguely recalled that her sister had some school problems but remembered few particulars. She wasn't worried about her parents' marriage. They had been quite understanding about her abdominal pain and were angry with the doctors for not having identified a cause yet. At times they got upset with her for not going to school, but they always seemed concerned when she was actually suffering. Her grandmother was the most adamant that she should return to school. Therefore, Betsy was not happy when she had to stay with her, except she liked it when she and the grandfather did fun things some afternoons. She also noted the grandmother's abdominal pain and the fact that the grandmother almost had surgery the previous year but was helped by medicine (although she still complained at times).

The parents and the child were told separately that further consultation was now necessary with the family doctor (the psychologist had already learned in a phone call to the family doctor that he was new to this family and thus did not know them well; so far, an extensive workup and specialist consultation had turned up nothing except the opinion that the pain was probably psychogenic). He would also need to contact the school. However, it appeared that Betsy was suffering from a separation anxiety disorder. Her abdominal pain was not uncommon and should be considered real and something that must be coped with. Multimodality intervention would be necessary, but there would be no medicine to begin with. The parents consented but were skeptical; they had already extensively considered whether any stress could be causing Betsy's problems but had come up with nothing. Betsy herself had little reaction except to express her desire to try anything that would get rid of the pain, even exploratory surgery.

The school guidance counselor was telephoned (the information from the English teacher's checklist was consistent with the parents' school history). The counselor indicated that Betsy had always been a rather shy, immature girl who was awkward with peers but had no major problem. The counselor knew of the past remedial reading and said that Betsy had always been an average student. Last year her usual grades dipped a little, and this year there were a couple D's (the reading help had been discontinued). Staff were surprised by her school absence since the holidays and would appreciate any guidance.

After this additional information was gathered and her case was reviewed again with the referring pediatrician, the family was seen again. Little had changed; the father had tried to insist that Betsy go to school, but that had not succeeded. The psychologist reconfirmed the diagnosis and explained that the initial thrust of treatment would involve collaborative work with the parents, Betsy, and school staff to ease the girl back into a normal school routine.

A meeting was arranged with all the school staff who worked with the girl. No significant new information emerged when the psychologist asked them for their observations. Betsy's type of absenteeism was relatively new to them; most absentees were actually truant, a situation that they knew how to handle better. They were more at a loss with this girl. The school had provided some home tutoring, but staff were now worried whether she could pass this school year. Most seemed sympathetic to her predicament, although some admitted they were annoyed that she wouldn't go to school and that her family couldn't make her.

The clinician summarized the important points of the girl's history and concluded with the diagnosis. He then reviewed the several possible diagnoses that could present as refusal to go to school in order to broaden the staff's appreciation of the complex differential diagnosis. Several questions were asked, and some staff began to recall past students who fit some of the other various diagnostic possibilities.

The child psychologist then stressed the seriousness of the girl's predicament and the need for collaborative effort to ease her back into school. He outlined a general plan: her hours in school would be extended gradually, and her missed work must also be introduced gradually, rather than overwhelming her all at once. The discussion continued on how to handle classmates' questions and reactions. Her need for positive reinforcement as she gradually resumed school was also emphasized. The psychologist also briefly described the therapy he would be conducting with Betsy and her parents, again emphasizing that collaborative effort was the key.

The guidance counselor volunteered to be the coordinator for the large number of junior high staff who had contact with her, an optimal choice because she already had a positive relationship with the girl. A second meeting between the psychologist and the staff was set in 1 week. The counselor and consultant would meet first for an hour to detail the plan. Then in the general meeting this plan would be thoroughly described and the psychologist would answer further questions from the staff. During this week the consultant also would have time to prepare the girl and her family to eventually meet with him and the counselor concerning the school arrangements. Finally, the psychologist reminded the counselor that at the next meeting they must further discuss two of Betsy's other needs: resumption of the help with reading and assistance with socialization skills. Both issues could well be affecting her current refusal to go to school.

Discussion:

1. The consultant was careful to do a comprehensive evaluation because of the several diagnostic possibilities: social phobia, conduct disorder, major depression, paranoid schizophrenia, panic disorder with agoraphobia, and avoidant disorder. Indeed, in this case, a reading disorder was identified that was not being sufficiently addressed in school; staff awareness of Betsy's learning disability was probably lost in the transition from grade school to junior high school. However, it appeared to be an exacerbating factor rather than the principal diagnosis.

2. The consultant used some of the initial meeting as an educational time to review the differential diagnosis. School staff typically

need knowledge of the different diagnoses that could cause school refusal; a review for school personnel was written by Strauss (1990). Such basic information can help teachers make more thorough observations and expedite early referral (especially to prevent the development of chronic school refusal and its increasing resistance to treatment). Such education can also aid staff in their initial handling of such situations. For example, if staff assume that they are dealing with early truancy when a student refuses to go to school, their approach could well be too confrontational and only exacerbate the situation.

3. The treatment of prolonged school refusal associated with separation anxiety disorder necessitates much collaborative work, with the therapist coordinating both family and school staff efforts. Thus, all school staff must understand the "game plan." A special, unhurried meeting to make sure that everyone is on the same page is preferable to a rushed review. Too often consultants assume that everyone understands the intervention design, when in reality staff may only partially understand the plan at the first discussion because they are easily distracted by their many other responsibilities. The additional meeting, as well as a school coordinator (always necessary after elementary school) to further supervise and answer questions, helps to guarantee a more successful reintroduction of the student back into school. Common antitherapeutic situations can be better avoided: a teacher overwhelming a student with the 2 months of homework that is due within the next 4 weeks; a nurse sending a student home because of the primary somatic complaint; sarcastic remarks by a teacher "welcoming" a student back; or the student sitting in the principal's office while the administrator scrambles to phone the family or doctor to learn what to do next.

4. Detailed descriptions of how to reintroduce children into school are not readily available, or they exist as case examples rather than techniques studied in homogeneous groups of children who refuse to attend school. Cognitive-behavioral techniques for use with anxious and school-refusal children and their families are available (Kendall et al. 1991), but research is still required to determine the most efficacious procedures (McReynolds et al. 1989).

Nevertheless, potentially useful approaches that include treatment in both school and home can be used (Blagg and Yule 1984; Yule et al. 1980). Blagg and Yule (1984) recommend the following: clarification of the child's problems, coordinated discussion and treatment by prepared school staff and parents, contingency plans to achieve maintenance of the child's return to school, gradual return to school with a capable escort, and sufficient follow-up, especially at vulnerable times (e..g., after Christmas vacation).

5. Frequently, students who refuse to attend school have chronic risk factors in school that must be addressed to decrease the chance that further stress will lead to relapse. In this case, the girl's need for remedial reading should be reevaluated. Also, her social skills, for which school intervention techniques are available, appear to require further assessment. Dodge (1989) summarized socialization steps that can be undertaken (e.g., in groups led by well-trained school staff): identification of problematic social tasks, identification of mechanisms related to social incompetence, improvement of social-cognitive skills, and improvement of behavior in problematic situations as well as overall social standing among peers.

C. SENIOR HIGH SCHOOL (CASE 3)

The following case example illustrates a consultant and a school staff facing the complex diagnosis and treatment planning for a depressed sophomore boy with learning disabilities:

David, a 16-year-old sophomore in his first year of high school, was seen by a child psychiatrist at school to be evaluated for a seriously emotionally disturbed (SED) class at the end of the first marking period. Referral material indicated that he was currently receiving no special programming. He was doing next to nothing in work and thus failing most subjects. Efforts to get him to work were usually met by defiance; sometimes he tried but soon got frustrated. He usually said little and rarely did anything the teachers asked of him. He also showed such growing irritability that his teachers were afraid that he was going to explode.

A review of past educational material disclosed that he had received speech therapy during the first three grades, as well as help for a problem with language comprehension. A reading problem was also identified in second grade for which he received remedial reading and then daily resource room help for the rest of grade school. His grades during elementary school were average, with more skills noted in math, art, and gym classes. Although easy frustration was noted, he was not considered to have a behavioral problem. He had some friends, but he often played by himself. The parents had not reported any major problems at home.

During his junior high years (seventh through ninth grade), David showed increasing problems. According to psychoeducational testing conducted by the school psychologist at the end of the past school year, his grades were falling. His learning disability (LD) resource room programming had continued and was almost half-time for most of ninth grade. During the testing he participated reasonably well. His verbal score on the Wechsler Intelligence Test for Children—Revised (WISC-R; Wechsler 1974) (subtests ranging from 7 to 9) was 18 points less than his performance score (subtests ranging from 8 to 12). Achievement testing showed him to be one grade behind in math and spelling and three grades behind in reading. Interestingly, he was slightly above his age in visual motor testing; indeed, he took that test with the most enthusiasm.

The actual consultation at school began with the team meeting. As the referral information indicated, the staff were worried about losing further ground with the boy. David came to school but did little work. He would daydream, sleep, or draw (with good renditions related to rock music themes). He still participated best in art, music, and gym classes, but his interest also appeared to be waning in those settings. The teachers were increasingly frustrated over their failed attempts to get him to work. Generally, he defiantly did nothing, and this year he had begun to swear occasionally at teachers and had even walked out of the room on a few occasions. The teachers sensed that he was giving up; several times he had wondered out loud what the worth of school was and had even mentioned dropping out. Outside the classroom, he associated with friends not unlike himself. Staff did not think these boys were getting into trouble in the community but were concerned about the possibility. He had been in a few scuffles at school, mainly verbal, and staff members were concerned about how angry he had appeared. These fights had occurred when some troublemakers called him or one of his friends "retard."

On follow-up questioning by the psychiatrist, staff admitted they were also concerned that David might be depressed, although they mainly saw anger; there had been no suicidal behaviors. During an initial session with a guidance counselor, he had broken down and cried, but then refused to come back. Some teachers were aware of his reading problem, whereas others reacted as if this was new information to them. The possibility of vocational school had been broached, but his parents had rejected that idea. They were cooperative but also quite insistent, especially his father, on his graduating with a "normal" education.

As the interview with David began, he did not look as though he was going to cooperate but soon became quite open. He had liked school more when he was younger but not anymore—he was just "knocking his head against the wall." He went because his parents made him, although he would like to graduate. But all the frustration was becoming more and more intolerable.

He knew he had a problem reading but did not know why and seemed unfamiliar with the concept of "learning disability." He generally understood people and conversed well. He did no reading outside the classroom. He basically "hung out," listening to music or playing video games. His friends shared similar interests and were not into substance use or trouble with the police; they wanted nothing to do with either.

When asked about his future, he shrugged but then admitted he was worried. Last summer he had done some work with his uncle, a carpenter, and was surprised how much he liked it; his uncle even thought he was good at it. He hadn't talked to his parents much about this. His mother seemed to appreciate his struggles in school. His father kept insisting that he try harder. Sometimes the father got very angry and would ground David or call him "lazy" or "dumb."

When the psychiatrist asked how all this was affecting his mood, David looked more sad. In recent years he hadn't been happy very often, except when he was with his friends. He was just constantly "blah" or irritable or unhappy. He did things but without much enthusiasm. He had rarely thought about suicide but rejected that as a solution. He often fell asleep worrying about the future but then generally slept through the night. Summers brought emotional relief.

Both parents came to their interview. Their observations were very similar to those of the school staff. School was now a trial for David. He was increasingly resistant to their pressuring or cajoling him to do homework. In contrast, he cooperated more with chores they asked him to do around the house. They did not see him as happy and were aware of general irritability. They were also concerned about his decreasing enthusiasm; he was even going out with friends less.

Their recollections of past history expanded the school history. His articulation problems had been quite severe and had brought a lot of kidding from peers. They recalled mention of language troubles, too, and the mother recalled that you often had to repeat yourself or make him say something back to you to be sure he understood. That was sometimes a problem even now. In contrast, he had always done better at sports but then had lost interest during junior high. He had always been a good artist, and they recalled last summer's job with the uncle as being a recent high point. He remained excellent at video games, usually better than his peers.

Although both parents could describe his learning problems (the mother more so than the father), they were not very conversant with the concept. The father admitted that he and a brother, and possibly their father, had school problems similar to David's. His own father had been "very strict" about school, and he was now glad of that. Indeed, he wished he had been less lazy and resistant because he might have gotten further ahead in life than being an auto mechanic. There was no history of affective disorders or suicidal behavior in either parent's family. Both parents recalled grounding and scolding their son for his school problems a lot in the past, feeling he must work harder. They had mellowed as he became older. They had always felt that he was trying, although less so over the past 2 years. Overall, no other major personal or family history was uncovered.

At the subsequent team meeting, the psychiatrist summarized the above interviews and then stated that David appeared to have chronic learning disorders (i.e., speech and language comprehension disorders and a reading disorder [not an uncommon combination]). Such children are at risk for psychiatric disorders, and it appeared the boy had developed a chronic depressive disorder (dysthymia), undoubtedly related to his chronic struggles in school. Now there was a vicious cycle. On the positive side, he had not developed serious conduct or substance use problems, he still seemed reachable, and he appeared to have some positive skills. Moreover, people still liked or felt for him, and his positive summer job experience was encouraging.

The psychiatrist suggested to the team that David needed several changes in school: instruction in alternative methods of information acquisition besides reading (where he may have reached a plateau), a different curriculum to make school a more meaningful experience, and treatment for his chronic depression. The staff suggested reevaluation by a reading specialist to reassess his LD needs (e.g., to consider the need for more visual learning aids). The staff had already considered vocational school, which had stimulated the boy's interest but which was rejected by the father. A current teacher worried that his present attitude toward work would not change quickly enough to allow him to succeed, especially because the vocational staff did not stand for much trouble from any student. However, the SED administrator at the meeting noted that an SED class had begun last year in the local vocational school and that some boys like David seemed to be responding to the combination of a vocational curriculum and an SED class. The SED teacher could continue David's LD programming while offering individual supportive counseling and serving as a resource for the vocational staff in regard to understanding the boy and his needs. Furthermore, group counseling on affective expression was also part of the SED curriculum. The psychiatrist further suggested that, whereas a vocational curriculum might create more positive school experiences, other positive school experiences possibly could be designed for him (e.g., drawing for the school newspaper, entering an art contest, and participating in seasonal decoration of the school).

The psychiatrist went on to note that this arrangement would probably satisfy both David and the parents. They might be encouraged about school becoming more meaningful for the boy, and the father would appreciate the continuance of "normal" schooling. However, the boy and his parents would need outside help to better understand his LD problems and cope with them more constructively, as well as to address his chronic mood disorder. The psychiatrist asked whether there was a local school psychologist with a part-time private practice who might best fill these needs. The team psychologist knew of some colleagues who dealt with such cases.

The crucial feedback was given to David and his parents together. The combination of disorders was described with a brief explanation about their connections. The whole family listened intently, nodding their heads at various times and asking a few appropriate questions. The treatment plan was then reviewed. At first the family was silent. David spoke first, saying he was skeptical but that he would like to give it a try because anything was better than now. The father remained concerned about the boy's future without "normal" schooling. The psychiatrist expanded on the concept of learning disorders and the need for a specialized curriculum to forestall further deterioration for the boy and to provide better preparation for his future. The mother began to cry and worry that they had approached him "all wrong." The psychiatrist consoled the mother, noting that such problems were difficult for children and their families to manage without help. The team school psychologist reassured them that a clinician who was attuned to their special needs was available.

The team psychologist then set up a meeting with the family to answer further questions and to develop a specific individualized education plan that they could sign. They all seemed inclined to approve this new direction, but it was clear that questions and skepticism remained. The psychiatrist repeated, in closing, that for David's sake the present situation could not continue, and this new plan represented a promising, defined option.

Discussion:

1. The educational history of this teenager with learning disabilities is much too common a scenario. A central question is whether he

received adequate programming during his earlier school years. Should he have been a full-time LD student, and how well were his complicated needs met? Were his mood difficulties more preventable? Once LD pupils with moderate to serious disabilities begin high school, they encounter further problems. Specialized resources generally become even more limited, and thus LD students are more on their own. The large number of teachers who deal with the student often have incomplete information about the student's ongoing LD problems, and some may not know at all. Thus, their ability to teach the pupil correctly is compromised, or they inadvertently confront the student with a confusing variety of styles or responses to his or her needs.

Finally, even though teachers know that a student has an LD, the student's defiance and their ensuing frustration may override their empathy or understanding. Thus, the poignant dilemma is encountered of teachers being angry at an LD student who is not working despite their awareness that the student often is incapable of keeping up with the work or the pace of the class.

2. Teachers are often aware that a student is depressed, but the consultant must ask them for this observation. Traditionally, a child referred for SED evaluation usually shows difficult externalizing behaviors. Relatedly, when teachers meet with a consultant, they frequently feel that it is proper to mention only externalizing problems. However, when the consultant asks about mood symptomatology, many staff are very forthcoming, whereas others are surprised that their colleagues perceive depression. Although many teachers have always been sensitive to depressive symptoms, more have now become better attuned, quite likely because of the extensive media attention focused on depression in recent years, especially the relationship between depression and suicide.

Relatedly, a consultant must not become lax. Although externalizing behaviors may be most apparent and thereby seemingly indicative of an externalizing diagnosis, thoroughness cannot be forgotten. Externalizing behaviors and diagnoses are commonly associated with affective disorders.

3. Parents of high school LD students can frequently provide valuable information about what their child actually experienced in

the past in relation to his or her LD. High school teachers generally cannot, and such information typically does not exist to much extent in the standard school records for students. In this boy's case, the parental information was helpful in understanding the probable genesis of his depression.

Also, in a younger student who may have an LD, classroom and testing data may be inconclusive. A good history of development from the parents can provide more solid evidence in that direction, much like the confirmatory facts supplied in this case.

4. In the treatment planning for this case, the psychiatrist served primarily as an organizer of the diagnostic thinking and as a catalyst for the staff's development of appropriate school interventions. In other words, the consultant recommended a therapeutic outline, and the staff was able to fill in the details based on local resources. This case is an excellent example of a collaboration where the consultant knew when to bow out and allow the staff to perform the educational functions for which they are trained.

5. A more necessary task for the consultant in this case was to explain the diagnoses and treatment plan to the boy and the parents in an effort to engage them in a working relationship with the school staff. The staff had previously been unsuccessful at developing this working relationship. Families will often accept a comprehensive treatment plan after contact with a consultant for several reasons. The family may assign the consultant greater authority because of his or her expertise in the situation, and thus be more accepting. They may feel the consultant is more knowledgeable on such matters, more so than the school staff, who are supposed to know only about teaching. Or the family may appreciate the consultant's thoroughness and the amount of time spent with them during the interview and feedback. Also, the family and school may already be in an emotional, adversarial relation about the student, and the neutrality and professionalism of the consultant are timely.

6. Importantly, the psychiatrist not only prescribed community intervention, but also was ready to follow through on its arrangement by having the school psychologist present at the family conference to aid with this referral. Indeed, a school staff member

should always be present at such feedback sessions. He or she should know exactly what the consultant tells the family, especially to prevent misunderstanding or future manipulation, and should serve as the ongoing contact with the family to advance the treatment plan. Also, this educator can further promote a positive working relationship between the family and the school.

7. What can school personnel do to more directly improve a student's depression? The treatment plan for this case included an affective training group within an SED class. Recent work has begun to demonstrate the success of groups that are specifically designed for depressed adolescent students and are led by properly trained school personnel (Kahn et al. 1990; Stark et al. 1989).

A reference that should prove valuable to school staff (especially school psychologists and guidance counselors), not only for basic education about depression in youth but also for potential intervention techniques, is Stark's *Childhood Depression: School-Based Intervention* (1990). A cognitive-behavioral approach is extensively described, including involvement of the family. Details are provided for conducting group therapy over 21 sessions. Topics of the sessions include self-reinforcement, self-monitoring of pleasant events, assertiveness training, social skills training, cognitive restructuring, problem solving, and attribution training.

The work of Stark and his colleagues represents some of the primary nonmedication, psychotherapeutic research in child and adolescent depression that currently exists in the literature. Subjects have been schoolchildren with depression, in contrast to the usual psychiatric outpatient or inpatient children. Stark emphasizes the need for future studies that combine treatment modalities, as well as research into the efficacy of the cognitive-behavioral approach with depressed children in both school and psychiatric settings.

8. Finally, how can the consultant deal with the emotionally charged question of whether this student received proper LD assistance during his school career? One danger is blaming the current school staff and thereby alienating them from participating, which would have been a disaster in this case because the staff proved extremely willing and constructive. A more constructive solution

might be to arrange a system consultation with key LD personnel, focusing on what went right and what went wrong in the handling of this case. Such interaction might lead to further system examination and subsequent improvements, depending on how favorably the educators regard the consultant. On the other hand, such a proposal could be rejected or halfheartedly accepted, as the implications of system changes are considerable and potentially very costly. Furthermore, the consultant might not have sufficient expertise or time to properly commit himself or herself to such a project.

D. SUMMARY

The three case consultations share six principles that are applicable for all school case consultation work:

1. *School information is necessary for any child psychiatric or psychological evaluation.* The more serious the problems in school, the more necessary is an actual meeting with all school personnel involved with the child in question. Such an initial meeting can promote a collaborative relationship for comprehensive treatment.

2. *Knowledge of school environments is vitally important, not only to understand what students experience, but also to appreciate the realities faced by the educational staff.* Such information is required to ask staff intelligent questions to gain their valuable information about a pupil's actual functioning in school. Moreover, when school intervention is necessary, such understanding will assist the consultant in the collaborative development of a realistic, practical treatment plan that the staff is likely to understand and carry out.

3. *Work with school personnel should always be understood as collaboration among professionals.* Although a consultant may propose an optimal comprehensive treatment plan, the actual intervention steps for the school should be developed by the whole team. The educators are the ones who must deliver the treatment in the classroom. Optimally, school intervention should be implemented,

monitored, and supervised by appropriate school personnel. Thus a consultant's role in classroom intervention is limited. Consultants are often asked to be God, when in reality school personnel must accomplish the task of intervention.

4. *A consultant should always be alert for chances to educate school personnel.* Thus, case consultations can often become consultee or system consultations that affect greater numbers of students. Helping school staff or a school district to develop its approaches to the several major child and adolescent diagnoses that it typically faces can have considerable importance.

5. *Treatment advice to school personnel,* unless a consultant already knows that they have high levels of understanding and skill, *should never be provided briefly* (e.g., at the end of a consultation). That would be analogous to teaching parent training to the parents of an ADHD child in the last 20 minutes of the evaluation time and expecting them to fully comprehend. Furthermore, the issue often is not only to educate a teacher, but also to develop the school's resources.

6. *Without direct knowledge of the student and family, consultants should be cautious about undertaking consultations that involve assisting a teacher or staff with a case that they present for discussion.* A consultant may assume that he or she understands the case sufficiently to help the staff, but beyond a teacher's summary may be complexity—as demonstrated in the above case examples. Incorrect diagnosis can lead to the wrong treatment approach and subsequent failure, which may then reduce the consultant's credibility in the eyes of the educators. Often it may be better to discuss a general type of student if this form of consultation is undertaken.

E. REFERENCES

Achenbach TM: Manual for the Child Behavior Checklist/4-18 and Profile. Burlington, VT, Department of Psychiatry, University of Vermont, 1991a

Achenbach TM: Manual for the Teacher's Report Form and Profile. Burlington, VT, Department of Psychiatry, University of Vermont, 1991b

Barkley RA: Attention Deficit Hyperactivity Disorder: A Handbook for Diagnosis and Treatment. New York, Guilford, 1990

Blagg NR, Yule W: The behavioral treatment of school refusal: a comparative study. Behav Res Ther 22:119–127, 1984

Braswell L, Bloomquist ML: Cognitive-Behavioral Therapy With ADHD: A Child, Family and School Model. New York, Guilford, 1991

Breen MJ, Altepeter TS: Disruptive Behavior Disorders in Children: Treatment-Focused Assessment. New York, Guilford, 1990

Dodge KA: Problems in social relationships, in Treatment of Childhood Disorders. Edited by Marsh EJ, Barkley RA. New York, Guilford, 1989, pp 222–246

Hawthorne Educational Services: The Attention Deficit Disorders Intervention Manual, School Version. Columbia, MO, Hawthorne Educational Services, 1989

Hinshaw SP, Erhardt D: Attention-deficit hyperactivity disorder, in Child and Adolescent Therapy: Cognitive-Behavioral Procedures. Edited by Kendall PC. New York, Guilford, 1991, pp 98–130

Kahn JS, Kehle TJ, Jenson WR, et al: Comparison of cognitive-behavioral, relaxation, and self-modelling interventions for depression among middle-school students. School Psychology Review 19:196–211, 1990

Kendall PC (ed): Child and Adolescent Therapy: Cognitive-Behavioral Procedures. New York, Guilford, 1991

Kendall PC, Chansky TE, Freidman M, et al: Treating anxiety disorders in children and adolescents, in Child and Adolescent Cognitive-Behavioral Procedures. Edited by Kendall PC. New York, Guilford, 1991, pp 131–164

McReynolds RA, Morris RJ, Kratochwill TR: Cognitive-behavioral treatment of school-related fears and anxieties, in Cognitive-Behavioral Psychology in the Schools. Edited by Hughes JN, Hall RJ. New York, Guilford, 1989, pp 434–465

Pfiffner LJ, Barkley RA: Educational placement and classroom management, in Attention Deficit Hyperactivity Disorder: A Handbook for Diagnosis and Treatment. Edited by Barkley RA. New York, Guilford, 1990, pp 498–539

Stark KD: Childhood Depression: School-Based Intervention. New York, Guilford, 1990

Stark KD, Best LR, Sellstrom EA: A cognitive-behavioral approach to the treatment of childhood depression, in Cognitive-Behavioral Psychology in the Schools. Edited by Hughes JN, Hall RJ. New York, Guilford, 1989, pp 389–433

Strauss CC: Anxiety disorders of childhood and adolescence. School Psychology Review 19:142–157, 1990

Wechsler D: Wechsler Intelligence Scale for Children—Revised. New York, Psychological Corporation, 1974

Yule W, Hersov L, Treseder J: Behavioral treatment in school refusal, in Out of School: Modern Perspectives in Truancy and School Refusal. Edited by Hersov L, Berg I. New York, Wiley, 1980, pp 267–302

Zentall SS: Self-control training with hyperactive and impulsive children, in Cognitive-Behavioral Psychology in the Schools. Edited by Hughes JN, Hall RJ. New York, Guilford, 1989, pp 305–346

CHAPTER EIGHT

Current Consultation Needs of School Systems

Richard E. Mattison, M.D.
Anthony Spirito, Ph.D.

This chapter focuses on system consultations commonly requested by school staff: identification of psychiatric disorders, management of suicidal behavior, primary prevention of contemporary problems, and delivery of psychological care in the school setting. Recent literature that bears on these issues is reviewed to help consultants reinforce the advice they give to schools. Indeed, these topics were selected because of their current importance to educators and the growing availability of objective reports on these topics.

A. IDENTIFICATION OF PSYCHOPATHOLOGY

School personnel are frequently confronted with children who demonstrate classroom dysfunction. They must then decide whether referral for evaluation or intervention, or both, is necessary. The training received by educational staff to help them make such decisions is variable and too often subjective (Pianta 1990); indeed, consultants are often asked for guidelines.

Empirical instruments may prove to be useful aids for school staff who deal with referral questions. They are economical, efficient, and familiar to many educators. In a report that should prove highly inter-

161

esting to educators, McConaughy and Achenbach (1989) described how a battery of checklists could prove helpful in the evaluation of a student for potential placement in a severely emotionally disturbed (SED) class. They discuss both the instruments and a protocol, and provide a case illustration.

In this section we review other recent work that may assist school staff in the identification of students who require intervention. Discussion focuses on the general determination of psychopathology that requires further evaluation or intervention, as well as on the specific identification of attention deficit and depressive disorders.

1. General Disorders

One research group has been developing a screening protocol to identify elementary students at risk for externalizing or internalizing disorders. Walker and Severson of the Oregon Research Institute have been investigating the potential of their Systematic Screening for Behavioral Disorders procedure (Walker and Severson 1990; Walker et al. 1988). In this multiple gating model, children in a grade school class could be screened in the following manner. First, the teacher ranks all the students with externalizing and internalizing behavioral problems (which are operationally defined). In the second stage, the top three children for both dimensions are further assessed by the teacher's completion of two instruments (with established psychometric properties): a checklist to indicate the presence or absence of critical behaviors and a measure to indicate the frequency of specific adaptive or maladaptive behaviors. Third, the students who meet or exceed the cutoff scores for both these instruments are then directly observed (according to prescribed instructions) in class for academic engaged time and in free play for peer interaction. Children who meet or exceed the cutoff criteria for one or both of these observational measures are then referred for further evaluation or treatment, or both.

This procedure has been carefully developed, and the findings thus far are quite promising. The developers hope that additional refinement will result in a screening protocol that may be used to identify children at risk for behavior problems, much as schools now screen for hearing or visual problems. Their emphasis is on identification as early as possible to allow timely intervention.

Related research has begun to focus on the identification of the level of intervention required by students with clear behavioral dysfunction in school, particularly those students in need of evaluation for SED placement. As a first step, Mattison and Gamble (1992) have shown significant differences between the scores of SED boys aged 6–11 years and the scores of boys who are psychiatric outpatients or who belong to the general population on the teacher and parent behavior checklists by Achenbach and Edelbrock (1983, 1986). This study also demonstrated the serious levels of dysfunction of SED boys in both the school and home environments: mean T scores were generally near to or greater than 70 (two standard deviations above the mean), with teacher ratings higher than parent ratings.

Once these basic differences were shown, the next step was to develop a procedure to help educators use teacher and parent checklist scores as one means of indicating that a child needs referral for community mental health or SED evaluation. Mattison and his colleagues have been investigating such a protocol (manuscript in preparation). Preliminary analyses of the teacher and parent checklists developed by Achenbach and Edelbrock suggest that the Total Problem scales of both checklists are the primary scales, in terms of accuracy and simplicity, for identifying at-risk students. Probability tables have been constructed so that educators can determine whether a boy's teacher and parent checklist scores indicate that he is in need of community services or referral for SED class consideration.

This procedure is viewed as a supplement to assist school personnel in their crucial decision-making about boys with behavioral or emotional dysfunction in school. Other factors may be equally or more important for educators to consider in determining the level of intervention required by a student. However, this line of investigation further shows the promise of objective instruments that can be used by school staff to assess the psychopathology they encounter in so many students.

2. Attention-Deficit Hyperactivity Disorder (ADHD)

As school personnel strive to deal more effectively with the problem of ADHD children, the question of how to identify ADHD may be posed to school consultants by school personnel. Currently, no protocol exists for the mass screening of ADHD in schoolchildren; thus, the issue is the proper evaluation of individual students. Although many children are referred to community professionals for the possible diagnosis of ADHD, many other students are referred first to school psychologists for the same diagnostic consideration. Thus, a school psychologist may request advice from a consultant on the diagnostic workup for ADHD, or a group of school psychologists or a school district may want consultation on how to standardize their approach to the diagnosis of ADHD.

Reviews on the assessment of children for ADHD have begun to appear in school journals (Guevremont et al. 1990; Schaughency and Rothlind 1991). More comprehensive information can be obtained by school personnel in the specific chapters on assessment in the books by Breen and Altepeter (1990) and especially Barkley (1990).

The consensus on proper assessment is a multimethod, multiobserver approach. The cornerstone is interviews of not only the parent(s) and the student, but also of the teacher(s). The use of structured clinical interviews is being encouraged to allow exploration of the symptoms that are the DSM-III-R criteria (American Psychiatric Association 1987) for ADHD. Although such an interview of teachers does not currently exist, Breen and Altepeter (1990) have proposed a general model. The major headings for their clinical interview of teachers are as follows: rationale for referral and overview of behavior problems, medical background and implications, cognitive issues, social interactions, general emotional state, interventions, child strengths, and questions regarding behavior questionnaires.

The information from the interviews is supplemented by more empirical data from behavioral questionnaires completed by parents and teachers and from specific psychological tests. These instruments can better address the issue of severity because of their normative bases, and they can provide objective baselines to monitor the effects of intervention. No one battery has emerged; school psychologists are probably best advised to experiment with different components until they find a set of instruments with which they are most satisfied. Relatedly, Barkley (1990) noted that the selection of a battery also depends on the purpose of the evaluation. In other words, the goals may vary: evaluation of an ADHD child aged 2–11 years versus an ADHD adolescent, evaluation of medication response versus effects of parent training, or evaluation of parent(s) adjustment.

Barkley and the other cited authors agree on a central point that consultants should stress when advising school psychologists on the evaluation of ADHD children—be comprehensive. The assessment of a pupil for ADHD is a complex undertaking, involving factors such as family, developmental levels, and comorbidity. Past standard workups used by school psychologists will no longer suffice (e.g., history from the teacher and an interview of the child, combined with intelligence, achievement, and projective tests). Although some school psychologists may be taken aback at the evaluation time and retraining that are involved, thoroughness is necessary. This more comprehensive understanding of an ADHD student should assist staff in planning more adequate school treatment and will likely increase the confidence and cooperation of the parent(s).

3. Depressive Disorders

When advising school psychologists about their evaluations for depressive disorders in children and adolescents, school consultants should use the same principles they use for ADHD. In other words, a comprehensive multiobserver approach is necessary, combining interviews and instruments. Recent literature on the assessment of childhood depression can prove useful, including articles by Kazdin (1987) and Reynolds (1990) and the diagnostic chapters in the recent book by Stark (1990) on school-based intervention for childhood depression.

Although the diagnostic approach may be the same for ADHD and depressive disorders, school psychologists have fewer available instruments to assess depressive disorders. Behavioral questionnaires and psychological tests for depression are not as well developed as those for ADHD; indeed, unlike instruments to assess ADHD, the most well-researched instruments for the assessment of childhood depression are self-report measures. Leading examples that have been used in school-based research are the Children's Depression Inventory (CDI; Kovacs 1979), the Reynolds Child Depression Scale (RCDS; Reynolds 1989), and the Reynolds Adolescent Depression Scale (RADS; Reynolds 1986a).

A procedure has been developed to screen for depression in large numbers of children and adolescents. Reynolds has proposed a multiple-stage model (Reynolds 1986b), which has been studied in preliminary research. A self-report depression questionnaire, like the CDI or the RCDS (or RADS), is administered to a large group of students. Within 1 month, the instrument is readministered to the smaller group of students who exceed the cutoff point at the first administration. Then, those students who exceed the cutoff scores at both time points are individually evaluated by clinicians. In his original field testing, Reynolds (1986b) reported that 18%–20% of a group of adolescent students scored in the depressed range after the first stage; after the third stage 7%–12% of the original group were identified by clinicians as clinically depressed. Stark (1990) reported that 16% of a group of children were identified as depressed after the first stage and overall approximately 5% were identified by the end of the clinical interviewing.

Although this model requires further research, it is promising. In addition, this multiple-stage approach might also be applied for screening large groups of students for ADHD. However, one practical caution should be emphasized when discussing mass screening for any psychopathology with school personnel. If increased numbers of students are identified as needing further evaluation or intervention, who will deliver these services? Currently, only about 20%–25% of the estimated 12%–15% of youth with psychiatric disorders receive psychological services (Institute of Medicine 1989); lack of trained professionals is one obstacle. Thus, a school district may like the idea of screening but be very hesitant about its implementation. One compromise would be more limited identification by the use of higher cutoff scores, thus attempting to guarantee that at least those students with the most severe conditions receive further attention.

B. SUICIDE PREVENTION

Over the last decade, high school staff have become increasingly aware of suicide and suicidal behavior in their students. Suicide prevention activities have become common in the educational setting. Thus, consultants may be asked to provide advice and recommendations to school personnel about prevention efforts that could be undertaken by the school, about students considered to be potentially suicidal or who have made a suicide attempt, and about the response of the school in the aftermath of a completed suicide. Issues associated with these topics are reviewed below. Two good general source books are *Suicide Prevention in Schools* (Leenaars and Wenckstern 1991) and *Suicide Intervention in the Schools* (Poland 1989). Recommendations at the systems level, such as developing school district policy and integrating school and mental health agencies in suicide prevention, can be reviewed in Davis et al. (1988) and Davis and Sandoval (1991).

1. Primary Prevention

Although suicide awareness programs in high schools have become very common, the effects of these programs on suicidal behavior are debatable. Those in favor of suicide awareness programs argue that education about suicide helps dispel myths existing in the student population, provides adolescents who are having significant suicidal ideation with enough information so that they might gain help for themselves, and provides both teachers and students with the type of information needed to act effectively if they encounter a suicidal student. These so-called "gatekeepers" who identify the suicidal student and make appropriate referrals are the key to a primary prevention program and thus need to be educated. Persons in favor of suicide awareness programs also believe that establishing these programs creates a suicide prevention "climate" in schools.

Those who oppose suicide awareness programs have several concerns. They believe that open discussion of the topic of suicide may lead to a "contagion effect" wherein suicide attempts actually increase. In other words, suicide awareness programs may "plant ideas" in the minds of students who have not previously been suicidal. These programs may inadvertently glamorize suicide for an adolescent, or they may arouse strong feelings that an adolescent cannot manage. Finally, suicide is described in a way that minimizes the level of psychopathology of a person who commits suicide.

The first decision a consultant must make is whether such educational programs regarding suicide are worthwhile. The empirical literature on this topic suggests that, at best, such programs are not particularly effective in changing attitudes and behavior (Spirito et al. 1988) or, at worst, they have slight negative effects (Shaffer et al. 1990). The American Association of Suicidology, on the other hand, strongly supports such educational efforts and believes that empirical studies to date have not measured very accurately or very well the positive effects that such educational programs have on students.

Assuming that such curricula are established in schools, the consultant may be asked to advise schools regarding what content and manner of presentation will be most effective in reaching students. First, the teacher of the course should make sure that the differentiation between suicide attempts and completed suicide is very clearly and repeatedly reinforced to students so that information about suicide attempters is not attributed to suicide completers. For example, the statement that a "normal" adolescent may *attempt* suicide under stress should not be interpreted as meaning that a "normal" adolescent may *commit* suicide under stress. Second, the risks attendant in attempted suicide (e.g., liver damage secondary to acetaminophen overdose and the possibility of inadvertent death from an overdose) need to be emphasized to students.

Third, it would be worthwhile for the consultant to evaluate the teacher's enthusiasm for and interest in teaching this subject. Often these curricula are assigned automatically to the science or health teacher. In such cases, the teaching can be poor and have a negative effect on students because of the teacher's lack of interest or other concerns. In these circumstances, the consultant might recommend that a new teacher be assigned.

Finally, the format of the suicide prevention curriculum should be considered. In many cases, this curriculum is presented as a separate portion of a health course. In isolation, only the topic of adolescent suicide is addressed, and coping skills and efforts to change behavior may be underemphasized. On the other hand, some curricula include discussions of mental health issues in general, and adolescent suicide is integrated into this topic area. These curricula often focus more on how to cope with different emotional stresses, including suicidal thoughts. Although the relative efficacy of these two types of teaching approaches has not been evaluated, the latter approach would appear to be more useful to adolescents.

A different approach to primary prevention of adolescent suicide in schools is screening the student body and then selecting at-risk students for more intensive evaluation. Some feel that such an approach, although more time intensive, is more helpful because resources will be directed toward those pupils in most need of intervention rather than toward the student body in general, the majority of whom have little need for prevention activities. Reynolds (1987) suggests that one way to screen adolescents is to administer the Suicide Ideation Questionnaire (which was administered to more than 6,000 high school students to develop appropriate norms and cutoff scores) and then to select those who report a high level of suicidal ideation. With this group approach, those who desire help but have difficulty asking for it may do so with the questionnaire because it is less threatening. Once these students are identified, the guidance counselor can interview them individually and report to the consultant, who then can make appropriate recommendations for further intervention. Administering such a scale en masse to a student body may be problematic to many principals and school boards. The argument might be raised that asking students to complete such a measure will "plant ideas" in the students' heads. Empirical data to support or refute this contention are lacking.

Another approach is to screen students individually with a brief in-person interview. Those at risk are then referred for further evaluation by mental health professionals. This approach has the advantage of allowing individual contact with students, which enables the interviewer to gauge the level of distress and whether intervention is necessary immediately. On the other hand, such an approach is more time intensive, and its practicality in many school systems may be questionable.

2. Secondary Prevention

Secondary prevention, as it is defined here, refers to the school's response to the student who appears suicidal or who has attempted suicide and returns to school. The consultant has several potential roles in regard to these students, including educating school professionals about suicidal signs in students, overseeing peer counseling services, and coordinating schools and community agencies in the treatment of suicidal students.

Recognition of the potentially suicidal student is a difficult task. The consultant must remember that many teachers are not particularly knowledgeable about adolescent emotional development. Consequently, training is necessary for these gatekeepers to recognize potentially suicidal students. The most practical way to conduct such training is through in-service programs for teachers. The consultant may wish to teach such an in-service program himself or herself. However, it is often a better use of the consultant's time to teach a core group of interested teachers the information necessary to detect suicidal students. In turn, the teachers are then available to work with other teachers within their own school or in the school system as a whole. Several of the sources referenced in this chapter (e.g., Poland 1989) provide helpful information about the type of knowledge that needs to be communicated to teachers in such in-service programs.

Some schools use fellow students as gatekeepers. These schools set up peer counseling programs designed to help identify and refer suicidal students. A faculty advisor usually oversees the program. When such a program is available in a school, the consultant will play a particularly important role in clinical decision-making about students at risk. These programs ultimately need a mental health professional available on short notice to make decisions that teachers will not have the knowledge or expertise to render. Thus, if the consultant recommends the establishment of such a peer counseling program, he or she must be aware that more intensive demands will be made on his or her time.

In either teacher-identified or peer-identified systems, the consultant may play an important role in helping the school to develop a written protocol for the identification of high-risk students. The consultant will also need to work with the school staff to establish a referral network within the community to assist those students in immediate need.

In the case of students who have attempted suicide, school officials can play several important roles. First, students who attempt suicide often are quite anxious about their return to school and their reception from other students. When a suicide attempter returns to school, a guidance counselor can assess his or her ability to handle the situation. Guidance counselors can also help these students problem-solve when difficult situations arise with other students.

Second, feedback to the community psychotherapist from school officials can be a valuable aid in treatment. In most cases, it will be up to the therapist to initiate such contact, and many times adolescents are reluctant to involve their schools in their treatment program. However, if school officials make contact with the adolescent's parents and offer their services to the community therapist, the opportunities to coordinate more effective care for the adolescent will increase. Such contact among the school, the parents, and the community treatment agency will require formulation of a policies and procedures protocol, such as that suggested by Kalafat and Underwood (1989). The consultant can play an important role in facilitating this communication between school and community because he or she has a foot in both camps. In other words, consultants are typically members of the mental health community and thus have opportunities to communicate with colleagues who are providing individual and family therapy to suicide attempters. As such, consultants can emphasize the potential value of coordination of treatment between the schools and community agencies.

Finally, it is important for school staff to realize that many adolescents receive very little psychiatric care after a suicide attempt. Many school officials assume that adolescents either are continuing in psychotherapy on a regular basis or have terminated psychotherapy because of significant progress. Yet too often adolescents and their families drop out of treatment or never receive any treatment after a suicide attempt. Thus, if there is regular communication between the school guidance counselor and the student, at least for the first few months after a suicide attempt, the school can be aware of whether ongoing treatment is being provided for the adolescent. By so doing, school officials can be especially attuned to suicidal cues in students who have attempted suicide but are no longer receiving any formal psychiatric care. In such cases, a guidance counselor may help the parents by offering to meet with the student on a more regular basis or by assisting the efforts of the parents to get the adolescent into treatment, or both. For example, guidance counselors might meet with a student to explain how treatment can be helpful, or they might work with ineffectual parents to clear up any obstacles interfering with their pursuit of treatment. Thus, consultants should promote effective communication among parents, schools, and community health professionals, as school staffs can play an invaluable role in ensuring that these adolescents are more closely monitored and receive ongoing counseling as needed.

3. Tertiary Prevention

In the context of the educational system, tertiary prevention refers to efforts directed toward prevention of further suicides in a high school after one or more suicides have occurred. *Postvention* refers to helping the survivors in the school cope with their distress. The manner in which schools respond to such situations differs substantially. For example, some schools may only observe a moment of silence, whereas other schools might provide release time for students to attend the funeral. A consultant may be asked to meet with teachers to address questions about how to handle the reactions of students in their classrooms and what cues they should be aware of to avert other suicides. Guilt is pervasive within a school after a completed suicide, and the consultant may find himself or herself dealing with it in many forms.

In most instances, the consultant may recommend that a more concerted effort be directed toward identifying and intervening with students at risk. This is particularly true after a cluster of suicides have occurred in the same school. Under these circumstances, communitywide intervention is indicated. A set of guidelines has been developed by the Centers for Disease Control (1988) regarding community responses to such crises. The consultant should review these guidelines for a better idea of the communitywide efforts that should be implemented after cluster suicides.

Brent et al. (1989) proposed one model for intervening with students in schools after a suicide. In this approach, guidance counselors and workers from local mental health agencies provide crisis intervention services for students at school. This intensive program in the schools is limited to approximately 3 weeks because of concern that a longer period of availability might actually exacerbate the problem by reminding students of the suicide for too long a time. Parents, teachers, and friends of the suicide victim are interviewed to determine the circumstances of the death. This information is important for identifying other students at risk for suicide; it also enables staff to provide objective information to the student body regarding the circumstances that surrounded the death. Many rumors and myths regarding the death often are promulgated throughout the student body, and such rumors should be dispelled to limit the probability of contagion. Students who were closest to the victim, who saw the victim alive last, or who may have witnessed the suicide may be particularly distressed and should also be interviewed.

Once these initial interviews have taken place and background facts about the suicides have been gathered, Brent and colleagues (1989) further recommend that a mental health professional meet with each homeroom class to discuss the suicides and the facts. Through such group meetings, high-risk students are identified for further intervention, including 1) those who directly request additional help, 2) those who are identified by another student in the classroom as needing emotional support, 3) those who appear visibly distressed during the classroom meeting, 4) friends of the victims, 5) anyone who attended the funeral, and 6) those with a prior psychiatric history. Once identified, these students are met with individually by a mental health professional, and a diagnostic interview is conducted to determine suicide potential. Other specific recommendations for consultants conducting postvention activities are reviewed in Lamb et al. (1991).

C. CONTEMPORARY PROBLEMS AND THEIR PRIMARY PREVENTION

A number of contemporary problems (such as substance abuse, AIDS, and teenage pregnancy) have had a substantial negative impact on schools. Other difficulties, such as violence, have been especially problematic for inner city and minority children. In addition to consulting in regard to students with such problems, mental health consultants may also be asked by schools to consult on the development or revision of primary prevention programs for such problems. Thus, consultants should be conversant with some of the most common approaches to prevention of these problems in school.

1. Programs for Minority Children

Prevention approaches have been designed to help minority students by affecting the social system of the school. One example is the School Development Program (SDP) in New Haven, Connecticut (Haynes et al. 1988). The SDP was designed to assist minority students and those from disadvantaged backgrounds in adjusting to school. A school planning and management team, led by the principal and composed of parents and teachers, analyzes the overall academic and social plan for the school. A mental health team addresses school climate issues as well as individual teacher and student problems. The parents program, a key component, involves parents in the planning of the school curriculum and activities. This program has been found to have a positive effect on school climate, as well as on the self-concept, behavior, and academic performance of students (Haynes and Comer 1990; Haynes et al. 1989).

2. Substance Abuse

Many different primary prevention programs for alcohol and other drug use have been developed and used in schools. Two major approaches to prevention have been implemented: 1) improving knowledge and awareness of the negative effects of alcohol and drugs and 2) behaviorally training students to resist peer pressures to use alcohol and other drugs (Botvin et al. 1989). Peer-led, as opposed to teacher-led, programs hold particular promise (Perry 1989). Although these programs are, in general, successful in improving knowledge and attitudes, they are less successful in changing behaviors (Kumpfer 1989). Guidelines for creating schools without drugs are also available for school administrators and parents (U.S. Department of Education 1989).

3. Violence

Violent behaviors have reached epidemic proportions in schools, particularly inner city schools. Minorities are much more likely than whites to be victims of violence in schools. Administrators are increasingly concerned about ways to decrease violence in schools. Thus, consultants may be called on to recommend approaches to violence prevention. The most well-known program is the Boston Youth Program Violence Prevention Curriculum developed by Prothrow-Stith (1986). This 10-session curriculum is designed for high school health classes and especially targets minority students. It provides facts about students' high risk for being victims of violence and teaches problem-solving skills specifically geared to violence (e.g., ways to avoid fights and alternatives to fighting). Other violence prevention programs are reviewed by the Carnegie Council on Adolescent Development (1991) and Prothrow-Stith (1986). All these programs are relatively new; thus, data regarding their effectiveness are only beginning to accumulate.

4. AIDS, Sexual Behavior, and Teen Pregnancy

In the last decade, AIDS prevention programs have been implemented in many schools across the country and are now mandated in most states. Although a component of these programs focuses on the risk of getting AIDS secondary to intravenous drug use, the major emphasis is typically on unprotected sexual behavior. Consequently, many parallels exist between sexuality education and AIDS education programs. Successful programs would result in a decrease in teenage pregnancy and human immunodeficiency virus (HIV) transmission. Studies demonstrate that improved knowledge does not typically cause changes in AIDS-related behavior (Hein 1990). Similar findings have been reported for school-based sex education programs (Kirby 1984).

Preventive education that starts before adolescents become sexually active appears to be more promising in reducing teenage pregnancy and is suggested for AIDS as well (Brown and Fritz 1988). Teaching methods that increase personalized concern about AIDS may have the most positive impact on AIDS-related attitudes and behavior. Techniques such as discussion sessions and visits by an HIV-positive individual are worth including in any curriculum (Ponton et al. 1991). The HIV Issues Committee of the American Academy of Child and Adolescent Psychiatry has produced two documents of value to consultants: the HIV/AIDS Information Sheet and the HIV/AIDS Issues Resource Guide, which provide helpful information about AIDS, including a list of resource materials for classroom use.

5. Identification of Students at Risk for Substance Abuse and Violence

In schools where substance abuse and violence are known to be prevalent, a consultant might suggest a schoolwide approach to identify at-risk students similar to the approach described for suicidal behavior. Substance abuse might be identified with a screening instrument entitled The Adolescent Drinking Index (Harrell and Wirtz 1987), a 24-item scale designed to screen for troubled adolescents who need more in-depth evaluation. This scale measures the severity of drinking problems in four areas: loss of control of drinking, social problems that result from drinking, drinking to relieve psychological problems, and physical problems that result from drinking. Normative data are available. Anger problems might be screened with the State-Trait Anger Expression Inventory (Spielberger 1988). This 44-item scale asks students to rate either the frequency or the intensity of their angry feelings and whether these feelings are expressed, suppressed, or controlled. Norms are available for high school students.

Alternatively, or in conjunction with the self-report screening of adolescents, teachers could be asked to identify students whom they think are substance abusers or who are angry or violent. Then these identified students could be assessed individually by guidance counselors for treatment needs. For such an identification program to be successful, a consultant should first educate teachers about signs of substance abuse and violence in their students (e.g., through in-service presentations).

D. SCHOOL-BASED CLINICS

Consultants should become aware of a relatively new movement that has the potential to increase the delivery of needed mental health services to students. School-based health centers and clinics have been growing in popularity since the 1980s. They arose amidst increasing concern about teen pregnancy and with the recognition that such programs might provide access to health care for large segments of youth who were receiving no such services. Mental health counseling was originally not a major component of such programs, but time has shown that almost 20% of students coming to school-based clinics use such counseling. Some information is emerging about the characteristics of the pupils seeking this counseling: depression, isolation, and stress are common. One survey revealed that 40% of such students had recently thought about committing suicide, and 18% had actually made an attempt (Center for Reproductive Health Policy Research 1989).

Basic knowledge about such programs is still in the early stages. Consequently, the literature thus far has primarily provided descriptions of various programs and patterns of usage. In general, school-based health centers provide medical screenings and treatment of minor problems at the school. Most offer varying services for family planning, pregnancy, and sexually transmitted diseases. Social services may be available, as well as counseling for personal or family problems. Staff size is not large, and the professionals often serve different roles.

Unfortunately, the mental health counselors in these clinics (typically from several disciplines, excepting psychiatry) usually perform only brief counseling or make referrals—which are very limited roles. In contrast, Adelman and Taylor (in press) have proposed six essential functions that would be desirable for a school-based mental health program: direct intervention with students, consultation with school staff, mental health education both in and out of school, outreach, resource identification and development, and networking. Thus, the mental health counselors would work directly not only with pupils, but also with school staff, parents, and community resources.

School-based mental health programs have great potential—not only in terms of service (especially to the many children and adolescents who would otherwise not have or seek such assistance), but also in terms of important research possibilities. For example, Adelman and Taylor (in press) note that the psychopathology and needs of adolescents might be better understood through investigations centered in school-based clinics, especially for underserved minority populations. Also, the effects of the multiple school-based psychosocial interventions might be better ascertained.

Consultants should familiarize themselves with such school-based programs that may now exist or could be established in their communities. School consultants would and should be natural contributors in several ways to school-based mental health clinics. In particular, their comprehensive overview of child psychopathology and their skills in working with and leading multidisciplinary teams would be invaluable in the crucial conceptualization and monitoring of such clinics. Properly developed programs could fill a tremendous void in the management of dysfunctional students—a void that individual consultants cannot fill alone and with which already overburdened school staffs cannot cope.

E. CONCLUSIONS

Ideally, school consultants should respond to questions with answers based, as much as possible, on evidence provided by research. Although the chapters cite empirical studies at times, most school consultation still clearly lacks any objective base. The need for collaborative research on school psychiatric issues has been receiving renewed emphasis, by both child psychiatrists and psychologists (Institute of Medicine 1989) and educators (Keogh 1990). In particular, the Institute of Medicine report stressed, "Connections between school programs and other disciplines within the child mental health field are scant; little advantage has been taken of research opportunities within such settings" (p. 167).

Hopefully, future chapters on school consultation will have a growing scientific basis. The current chapters suggest some directions (e.g., standard evaluation and consultation procedures and recommendations based on established proof). Most important, collaborative, professional working relationships between educators and child psychiatrists and psychologists are emphasized, because these relationships are the starting point for research.

F. REFERENCES

Achenbach TM, Edelbrock C: Manual for the Child Behavior Checklist and Revised Child Behavior Profile. Burlington, VT, Department of Psychiatry, University of Vermont, 1983

Achenbach TM, Edelbrock C: Manual for the Teacher's Report Form and Teacher Version of the Child Behavior Profile. Burlington, VT, Department of Psychiatry, University of Vermont, 1986

Adelman HS, Taylor L: Mental health facets of the school-based health center movement: need and opportunity for research and development. J Ment Health Adm (in press)

American Psychiatric Association: Diagnostic and Statistical Manual of Mental Disorders, 3rd Edition, Revised. Washington, DC, American Psychiatric Association, 1987

Barkley RA: Attention Deficit Hyperactivity Disorder. New York, Guilford, 1990

Botvin GJ, Schinke SP, Orlandi MA: Psychosocial approaches to substance abuse prevention: theoretical foundations and empirical findings. Crisis 10:62–77, 1989

Breen MJ, Altepeter TS: Disruptive Behavior Disorders in Children: Treatment-Focused Assessment. New York, Guilford, 1990

Brent D, Kerr M, Goldstein C, et al: An outbreak of suicide and suicidal behavior in a high school. J Am Acad Child Adolesc Psychiatry 28:918–924, 1989

Brown L, Fritz G: AIDS education in the schools: a literature review as a guide for curriculum planning. Clin Pediatr (Phila) 27:311–316, 1988

Carnegie Council on Adolescent Development: Life Skills Training: Preventive Interventions for Young Adolescents. New York, Carnegie Corporation, 1990

Center for Reproductive Health Policy Research: Annual Report: Evaluation of California's Comprehensive School-Based Health Centers. San Francisco, CA, Center for Reproductive Health Policy Research, Institute for Health Policy Studies, University of California at San Francisco, 1989

Centers for Disease Control: CDC recommendations for a community plan for the prevention and containment of suicide clusters. MMWR (Suppl S-6):1–12, 1988

Davis J, Sandoval J: Suicidal Youth: School-Based Intervention and Prevention. San Francisco, CA, Jossey-Bass, 1991

Davis J, Sandoval J, Wilson M: Strategies for the primary prevention of adolescent suicide. School Psychology Review 17:559–569, 1988

Guevremont DC, DuPaul GJ, Barkley RA: Diagnosis and assessment of attention deficit-hyperactivity disorder in children. Journal of School Psychology 28:51–78, 1990

Harrell A, Wirtz P: Adolescent Drinking Index: Professional Manual. Odessa, FL, Psychological Assessment Resources, 1987

Haynes NM, Comer JP: The effects of a school development program on self-concept. Yale J Biol Med 63:275–283, 1990

Haynes NM, Comer JP, Hamilton-Lee M: The school development program: a model for school improvement. Journal of Negro Education 5:11–21, 1988

Haynes NM, Comer JP, Hamilton-Lee M: School climate enhancement through parental involvement. Journal of School Psychology 17:87–90, 1989

Hein K: Lessons from New York City on HIV/AIDS in adolescents. N Y State J Med 90:143–145, 1990

Institute of Medicine: Research on Children and Adolescents With Mental, Behavioral and Developmental Disorders. Washington, DC, National Academy Press, 1989

Kalafat T, Underwood M: Lifelines: A School-Based Adolescent Suicide Response Program. Dubuque, IA, Kendall/Hunt, 1989

Kazdin AE: Assessment of childhood depression: current issues and strategies. Behavioral Assessment 9:291–319, 1987

Keogh BK: Narrowing the gap between policy and practice. Except Child 57:186–190, 1990

Kirby D: Sexuality Education: An Evaluation of Programs and Their Effects. Santa Cruz, CA, Network Publications, 1984

Kovacs M: Children's Depression Inventory. Pittsburgh, PA, School of Medicine, University of Pittsburgh, 1979

Kumpfer K: Prevention of alcohol and drug abuse: a critical review of risk factors and prevention strategies, in Prevention of Mental Disorders, Alcohol and Other Drug Use in Children and Adolescents (DHHS Publ No ADM 89-1646). Edited by Shaffer D, Philips I, Enzer N. Washington, DC, U.S. Government Printing Office, 1989, pp 309–372

Lamb F, Dunne-Maxim K, Underwood M, et al: Postvention from the viewpoint of consultants, in Suicide Prevention in Schools. Edited by Leenaars AA, Wenckstern S. New York, Hemisphere, 1991, pp 213–230

Leenaars AA, Wenckstern S (eds): Suicide Prevention in Schools. New York, Hemisphere, 1991

Mattison RE, Gamble AD: Severity of SED boys' dysfunction at school and home: comparison with psychiatric and general population boys. Behavioral Disorders 17:219–224, 1992

McConaughy SH, Achenbach TM: Empirically based assessment of serious emotional disturbance. Journal of School Psychology 27:91–117, 1989

Perry C: Prevention of alcohol use and abuse in adolescence: teacher vs. peer-led intervention. Crisis 10:52–62, 1989

Pianta RC: Widening the debate on educational reform: prevention as a viable alternative. Except Child 56:306–313, 1990

Poland S: Suicide Intervention in the Schools. New York, Guilford Press, 1989

Ponton L, DiClemente R, McKenna S: An AIDS education and prevention program for hospitalized adolescents. J Am Acad Child Adolescent Psychiatry 30:729–734, 1991

Prothrow-Stith D: Interdisciplinary interventions applicable to prevention of interpersonal violence and homicide in black youth, in Report of the Secretary's Task Force on Black and Minority Health, Vol 5: Homicide, Suicide, and Unintentional Injuries. Washington, DC, U.S. Public Health Service, 1986, pp 227–244

Reynolds WM: Reynolds Adolescent Depression Scale. Odessa, FL, Psychological Assessment Resources, 1986a

Reynolds WM: A model for screening and identification of depressed children and adolescents in school settings. Professional School Psychology 1:117–129, 1986b

Reynolds W: Suicide Ideation Questionnaire. Odessa, FL, Psychological Assessment Resources, 1987

Reynolds WM: Reynolds Child Depression Scale. Odessa, FL, Psychological Assessment Resources, 1989

Reynolds WM: Depression in children and adolescents: nature, diagnosis, assessment, and treatment. School Psychology Review 19:158–173, 1990

Schaughency EA, Rothlind J: Assessment and classification of attention-deficit hyperactive disorders. School Psychology Review 20:187–202, 1991

Shaffer D, Vieland U, Garland A, et al: Adolescent suicide attempters: response to suicide-prevention programs. JAMA 264:3151–3155, 1990

Spielberger C: State-Trait Anger Expression Scale: Professional Manual. Odessa, FL, Psychological Assessment Resources, 1988

Spirito JA, Overholser J, Ashworth J, et al: Evaluation of a suicide awareness curriculum for high school students. J Am Acad Child Adolescent Psychiatry 27:705–711, 1988

Stark K: Childhood Depression: School-Based Intervention. New York, Guilford, 1990

U.S. Department of Education: What Works: Schools Without Drugs. (Copies available from National Clearing House for Alcohol and Drug Information, P.O. Box 2345, Rockville, MD 20852.) Washington, DC, U.S. Department of Education, 1989

Walker HM, Severson HH: Systematic Screening for Behavior Disorders. Longmont, CO, Sopris West, 1990

Walker HM, Severson HH, Stiller B, et al: Systematic screening of pupils in the elementary age range at risk for behavior disorders: Development and trial testing of a multiple gating model. Remedial and Special Education 9:8–19, 1988

FORENSIC CONSULTATION

Barry Nurcombe, M.D.

Section III: Forensic Consultation

Chapter Nine
The Law and the Legal System
    A. Nature and purposes of the law
    B. Sources of the law
        1. Constitutional law
        2. Statutory law
        3. Case law
        4. Administrative law
    C. The legislative process
    D. The court system
        1. Federal courts
        2. State courts
    E. Judicial proceedings
        1. Criminal proceedings
        2. Quasicriminal proceedings
        3. Civil court proceedings
        4. Administrative hearings
    F. Adjudication
        1. The rules of evidence
        2. Types of witnesses
        3. Standards of proof
        4. Judicial reasoning
        5. Case law and precedent
    G. Legal advocacy
    H. Summary
    I. Selected readings
    J. Table of cases
    K. References

Chapter Ten
Legal Issues Commonly Requiring Mental Health Consultation
    A. Child custody disputes
        1. Legal doctrines
            a. Maternal preference
            b. Best interests of the child

        c. Continuity of care

    2. Types of custody

        a. Single parent custody

        b. Joint parental custody

    3. Controversial issues

        a. Moral unfitness

        b. Parental mental illness or impairment

        c. Child's religion or race

        d. Child's preference

        e. Siblings

        f. Substantial change of circumstances

        g. Relocation of the custodial parent

        h. Allegations of sexual abuse

        i. Rights of grandparents

        j. Child snatching

        k. Lesbian parents

    4. Effects of divorce on children

  B. Child maltreatment

    1. Legal doctrines

        a. Parens patriae

        b. Best interests of the child

    2. Situations giving rise to intervention

        a. Physical abuse

        b. Neglect and abandonment

        c. Sexual abuse

        d. Emotional abuse

        e. Educational and medical neglect

        f. Parental incapacity

    3. Child protection hearings

    4. Research into the effects of sexual abuse on children

  C. Civil liability

    1. Legal doctrines

        a. Definitions

        b. Elements of a negligent tort

        c. Compensation

        d. Negligent infliction of emotional distress

Chapter Eleven
The Forensic Evaluation
-   A. The expert witness
-   B. The evaluation
    1. Initial contact
    2. Initial interview
    3. Evaluation questions
        a. Diagnosis
        b. Severity
        c. Pattern
        d. Causation
        e. Preexisting condition
        f. Perpetuation
        g. Prognosis
    4. Evaluation procedures
    5. Elucidating the questions
        a. Diagnosis, severity, and pattern
        b. Causation
        c. Aggravation
        d. Perpetuation
        e. Prognosis and recommendations
-   C. Records
-   D. The forensic evaluation report
-   E. Summary
-   F. Selected readings
-   G. Table of cases and laws
-   H. References

Chapter Twelve
Giving Testimony as an Expert Witness
-   A. The pretrial conference
-   B. Preparing to be deposed or to give testimony in court
-   C. Deposing
-   D. Testifying
    1. Preparing to testify
    2. Qualification
    3. Direct examination
    4. Cross-examination

CHAPTER NINE

The Law and the Legal System

Barry Nurcombe, M.D.

M ost clinicians dread the arrival of a subpoena. Adrift in the halls of justice, frustrated by the law's delay, and insulted
when their credentials are impeached, they are likely to conclude
that the adversary system obscures the truth and that the rules of
evidence impede a balanced exposition of the case. Lawyers, for
their part, are dubious of psychiatrists, psychologists, and social
workers. What is the difference between them? To which "school"
do they belong? Isn't mental illness a myth (as they were told in their
college sociology courses)? Aren't psychiatrists the agents of a cor-
rupt State that conspires to sequester dissidents and eccentrics (as
they read in the delirious sixties)? Shouldn't mental health experts
have medical qualifications? Aren't psychiatry and psychology "in-
exact" or "soft" sciences, flaccid enough to be bent toward any point
of view? Moreover, lawyers often feel that clinicians are inclined to
be gulled by everything their patients tell them and are seemingly
oblivious as witnesses to the bias and conflicts of interest that ensue.

The increasing involvement of mental health clinicians in forensic
matters has met with scathing criticism from within psychology itself.
Faust and Ziskin (1988) asserted that clinical judgment is suspect
with regard to such matters as diagnosis, credibility, competence, potential for violence, and an offender's mental state at the time of a
crime. They contended that there is no convincing evidence that cli-

nicians with years of experience are any better than novices or even laypersons. Furthermore, they argued, scientific data are properly presented in an actuarial, probabilistic form unsuitable for the black-and-white requirements of the courts. They concluded that mental health experts lack sufficient certitude to give reliable opinions; therefore, until research yields better methods and more relevant and solid information, clinicians should recuse themselves from the forensic arena.

From the viewpoint of a lawyer, Morse (1978) criticized mental health experts on the grounds that lay people are quite competent to decide whether defendants are insane or incompetent. He further contended that legal judgments have to do with morality and social policy, which are outside the province of clinical expertise; clinicians usurp the responsibility of judges and juries when they pronounce opinions on such matters (see Chapter 11).

In answer to these criticisms, Slobogin (1980) and Melton et al. (1987) argued for limited forensic involvement by mental health experts. They agreed with Morse that clinicians should refrain from giving opinions concerning ultimate issues (e.g., competence to stand trial, exculpation by reason of insanity, civil liability, and the best interests of a child). However, if clinicians are properly qualified by reason of both general and forensic training and experience, if they appreciate the legal questions at issue in the case, if they employ established techniques of known reliability and validity, and if they elicit clinical data thoroughly and weigh its significance impartially, then they can throw light upon many of the legal issues that the courts must examine in rendering final judgment. The current trend, in any case, is to admit mental health testimony and to leave it to the judge or jury to decide whether the probative merit of the evidence outweighs its unreliability, irrelevance, or inefficiency. Psychiatric diagnosis, for example, is no less accurate than radiological diagnosis. Even psychodynamic explanations linking early experience with later behavior, although admittedly speculative, can broaden the court's perspective.

Notwithstanding the contemporary minefield of ethical, procedural, and communicative problems, the desire of the courts for expert opinion has induced more and more clinicians to become involved in forensic cases. A small but growing band of child psychiatrists, psychologists, and social workers are founding a new subspecialty. Unquestionably, the most reliable and valid forms of assessment are still being forged, and the degree of certitude associated with different conclusions needs clarification. Nonetheless, scientific evidence concerning the outcome of different forms of custody and permanency planning, the psychosocial consequences of accidental trauma, the results of physical and sexual abuse, and the forms and etiology of juvenile crime are topics of great social, legal, and scientific importance. The law is changing, particularly in the fields of children's rights, child custody, and child protection. Legislators and lawyers need help if they are to frame and interpret laws that take into account the developmental needs of children and the special requirements of the physically, educationally, and mentally impaired.

It is essential that clinicians involved in legal proceedings be familiar with the nature and sources of the law, the conduct of legal proceedings, and the proper manner of communicating with lawyers. Otherwise, their forensic evaluations will miss the mark. This chapter and the next three introduce the clinician to these matters.

A. NATURE AND PURPOSES OF THE LAW

The law is an assemblage of authoritative constitutions, policies, procedures, regulations, statutes, and precedents, implemented by authorized people and institutions. The law sets limits on the extent to which the state can infringe on private rights, defines the rights and obligations of citizens with regard to each other and the State, stipulates the sanctions to be enforced by the State on those who infringe on its rules, and regulates the proceedings by which disputes or charges are settled or disposed of.

Let us examine this definition point by point. First of all, it is important to appreciate that the law is an assemblage formed by successive depositions of ideas from custom, precedent, and legislation. Although conservative, the law is dynamic and evolving, for the past is constantly reinterpreted in response to contemporary needs. In *Roe v. Wade* (1973), for example, the Supreme Court reinterpreted the Bill of Rights and the Fourteenth Amendment to the Constitution by ruling that, during the first trimester of pregnancy, a woman's right to privacy is paramount and may not be preempted by the state's legitimate desire to regulate abortion. This decision has been the subject of continuing debate.

The law is authoritative; in other words, it has been invested with the power to regulate. In its regulatory function, the law is derived from the regulations and policies of administrative bodies (such as Departments of Child Welfare), from the statutes enacted by state legislatures, from procedural rules (e.g., the federal rules of evidence), and from precedents in the form of case law (see section B3, "Case Law").

The agents of the law—legislators, police, court officials, judges, and attorneys—are authorized by the people to frame the laws, keep the peace, apprehend alleged miscreants, operate the courts, try cases, and advocate for one side or the other in a dispute. In accordance with defined processes and limits, the courts are empowered to impose and enforce sanctions against those who have been found guilty of transgressing the law. These sanctions range from a reprimand, through the exaction of fines or the deprivation of liberty, to execution for a capital offense.

The law defines the obligations of citizens to the State and to each other (e.g., to pay taxes and to drive motor vehicles with due care for others). The federal and state constitutions define the people's rights by setting the limits within which law enforcement must operate if it proposes to alienate a citizen's basic liberties. In other words, the law must be enforced according to rules. For example, searches of citizens and the seizure of personal property must be warranted (or at the very least based on reasonable suspicion of wrongdoing). In criminal proceedings, the individual must be accorded due process; for example, in serious offenses the accused is afforded a public hearing, legal counsel, the right to confront and present witnesses, an impartial jury, and a judge who ensures that the case is fairly tried and who may not impose excessive punishment. Thus, as the law disposes of cases and settles disputes, it aims to do so consistently, impartially, justly, and mercifully.

American law pits one party against another in a formalized tug-of-war aimed to expose the arguments for and against each side. A trial is less an investigation than a demonstration, for it may not go beyond the evidence presented by the contending parties. Slovenko (1973) compared a trial to a game, because it reenacts a traumatic event to resolve it. Through this reenactment, society reasserts the primacy of its rules and gains mastery over incidents that disturb the peace. The elaborate, formalized procedures of the court are designed to hold passion at bay so that reason may prevail. From another viewpoint, Slovenko suggested, the courtroom is a dramatic stage on which good and evil, right and wrong, and protagonist and antagonist contend, in search of a verdict that will resolve their conflict. The theater of law, so to speak, stages morality plays that uphold the rules of society and demonstrate that justice will be done.

. Slovenko (1973) pointed out that law differs from science in several ways. Science is theoretical; law is practical. Science seeks to approximate the truth; law aims to resolve disputes. Science seeks accuracy through experiment and measurement; law attempts to get at the facts through mutual impugnment. A lawyer's duty is to advocate his or her client's case within a framework of professional ethics and law; a scientist's task is to advance knowledge of the formal relationships between things or events. The law honors ritual and bows to authority; science is skeptical of precedent. The law embodies and executes values; science strives to be value free. Slovenko emphasized the differences between law and science to clarify matters that frequently confuse clinicians who become caught in the crossfire of the courtroom. Naive clinicians may be affronted by the vigor with which cross-examiners question their qualifications, techniques, and opinions. They should not take such encounters personally, but, rather, should learn to appreciate them as the means by which the true quality of their testimony is tested.

B. SOURCES OF THE LAW

American law is derived from federal and state constitutions, from legislative statutes, from administrative regulations and ordinances, and from the precedents of case law.

1. Constitutional Law

The federal and state constitutions represent the people's view of the fundamental relationship between citizens and their government and the extent to which the State may infringe on individual liberty. The federal constitution consists of seven articles that set out the composition, election, sources of revenue, function, and powers of the Congress, the President, and the Supreme Court, together with the rights and obligations of the states toward the federal government. The powers of the federal government were originally limited by 10 amendments, known as the Bill of Rights. By 1988, the 10 original amendments had been expanded to 26. Of greatest significance to the mental health practitioner are the First, Fourth, Fifth, Sixth, Eighth, and Fourteenth Amendments. We will now consider how these amendments have been deemed to apply to minors.

The First Amendment prohibits the State from imposing an official religion, limiting free speech (unless there is a "clear and present danger"), curtailing the freedom of the press (except in matters of national security or obscenity), and preventing people from associating with each other (with specified exceptions). The relevance of the First Amendment to minors' rights was reviewed, for example, in *Tinker v. Des Moines Independent Community School District* (1969). In this case, The Supreme Court upheld the right of schoolchildren to wear black armbands as a protest against the Vietnam war, provided their protest was not aggressive, destructive, or disruptive of school discipline. On the other hand, in *Hazelwood School District v. Kuhlmeier* (1988), the Court upheld the right of school authorities to edit the style and content of a school newspaper, "so long as their actions were reasonably related to legitimate pedagogical concerns."

The Fourth Amendment concerns the right of the people to be secure in their persons, houses, papers, and effects. Warrants are required to enter and search private property and may be issued only on probable cause (see section F3, "Standards of Proof"), supported by oath or affirmation. This constitutional issue was debated in *In re TLO* (1983). In this case, a high school student appealed against an unwarranted search of her purse by school authorities (although drugs were in fact discovered). The Court ruled that the authorities had had probable cause for the search and seizure.

The Fifth Amendment prescribes grand jury indictment for capital or infamous crimes, proscribes double jeopardy and self-incrimination, and mandates due process and just compensation (if the State proposes to resume private property). Both the self-incrimination and the double-jeopardy clauses have been extended to minors (*In re Gault* 1967; *Kent v. U.S.* 1966).

The Sixth Amendment requires that, in criminal cases, the accused be provided with the following: a speedy, public trial; an impartial jury; information as to the nature and cause of the accusation; the right to confront and cross-examine accusers; the right to secure witnesses by subpoena; and the right to counsel. The clauses to do with the public nature of the trial and the right to confront witnesses are germane to the controversy concerning the legitimacy of screened or videotaped testimony for sexual abuse victims. In *Coy v. Iowa* (1988), The Supreme Court struck down an Iowa statute permitting the use of one-way screens, ruling that the interests of the victim did not outweigh the due process rights of the accused. However, the Court raised the possibility that the right to confrontation might be waived, on a case-by-case basis, "upon a showing of necessity." The protection of the child witness from psychological harm was described as a legitimate state interest that might, in particular cases, be shown to outweigh a defendant's Sixth Amendment rights.

The Eighth Amendment proscribes excessive bail, egregious fines, and cruel and unusual punishment. Juveniles have no right to bail. However, the right to be free of cruel and unusual punishment has been held to apply to inmates of a juvenile correctional institution who had been subject to solitary confinement and brutal methods of crowd control (*Morales v. Turman* 1971).

The Fourteenth Amendment protects the "privileges and immunities" of citizens and mandates due process and equal protection. The equal protection clause was the basis for the momentous civil rights decision against racially segregated schooling (*Brown*

v. Topeka Board of Education 1954). The right to privacy that un-
derpinned the Supreme Court's decisions concerning first-trimes-
ter abortion was derived from the privileges and immunities
clause of the Fourteenth Amendment (*Roe v. Wade* 1973). Earlier,
in *Griswold v. Connecticut* (1965), the right to privacy had been
held to emanate from the "penumbras" surrounding the Bill of
Rights and the Ninth Amendment. When a minor independently
seeks abortion, the court must balance her right to privacy against
the parents' right to bring up their children without interference
by the State and the State's legitimate interest in regulating abortion (e.g., *Bellotti v. Baird* 1979). The due process clause of the
Fourteenth Amendment has been held to apply to juvenile offenders (*In re Gault; Kent v. U.S.*).

2. Statutory Law

Statutes and ordinances are enacted by lawmaking bodies such
as Congress, state legislatures, and town councils in order to
change or advance the common law. Statutes define terms, par-
ticularize conditions, and authorize specified agents or agencies.
For example, all states have mental health acts that codify the
power of the government to abridge the liberty of citizens on the
grounds of mental illness. If statutory laws violate the terms of
the U.S. Constitution, they are likely to be contested in federal or
state courts. If state law and the U.S. Constitution conflict, the
U.S. Constitution will prevail.

3. Case Law

Criminal law concerns crimes against the State, whereas civil law
applies to disputes between private citizens. The common law is
an inductively derived collection of customs and legal precedents that evolved from English law. Common law and statutory
law are continually reinterpreted by the courts as case law. To
this extent, case law is judge-made law. Within a particular state,
the holdings of an appellate court regulate lower courts. Outside
that state, the rationale for an appellate court's decision may be

quoted by an attorney or judge to support or rebut a particular argument, but the opinion has no binding authority beyond its state of origin. Thus case law interprets legal principles and statutes by applying them to particular cases, whereas the doctrine of stare decisis (precedent) favors consistency by ensuring that, if a similar point is at issue, a prior judicial holding will become binding in the same court or in courts of equal or lower rank.

The traditional case-by-case construction of legal doctrine has been under attack in recent years. On the one hand, judges are seen as "filling the open spaces in the law," "legislating between the gaps," and gradually adapting established doctrine to new conditions. On the other hand, judges have been criticized for imposing their biases on the citizenry, thus usurping the proper function of elected legislators. The continuing debate over *Roe v. Wade* illustrates the point. Some see the articulation of a right to privacy as a landmark; others regard it as an improper interpretation of the Constitution and the imposition of personal prejudice on the community by officials who do not have to answer to the electorate.

Some of the most influential judicial decisions have been rendered in class action suits. Class action suits may be brought in state or federal courts. In such cases, a single suit is advocated on behalf of many people with similar grievances (e.g., *Roe v. Wade, Brown v. Topeka Board of Education*). Class actions were much favored by activists between 1950 and 1975; however, more restrictive federal rules and reduced funding for public legal agencies have diminished the frequency of this kind of case.

4. Administrative Law

Administrative agencies operate at federal, state, and local levels. They are empowered by the legislature to issue regulations in accordance with which they implement the intent of legislation. For example, the Internal Revenue Service is regulated by its own set of principles and precedents; and child welfare departments must work within a regulatory environment. The regulations by which an agency must abide are procedural (i.e., the methods according to which it should operate), interpretive (i.e., the guidelines by which the agency must interpret its mandate), and substantive (i.e., the actual rules formulated by the agency in accordance with its mandate). If conflict arises, statutes supersede administrative regulations, and federal regulations supersede state law.

In fulfilling its mandate, an agency may have the authority to assume the custody of a child (e.g., a child welfare agency may remove a child from a neglectful home), to prosecute and adjudicate (e.g., the Internal Revenue Service holds adversarial hearings with counsel, witnesses, and judge), and to make rules (e.g., the Department of Health and Human Services promulgated rules and guidelines based on Public Law 98-457—the "Baby Doe" regulations). The courts may be called on to interpret an agency's regulations. For example, at one point in the "Baby Doe" case (*American Academy of Pediatrics v. Heckler* 1983), a federal court held that an "interim final regulation" promulgated by the Secretary of Health and Human Services was "arbitrary and capricious" and that the department was acting ultra vires.

C. THE LEGISLATIVE PROCESS

In contrast to federal judges, legislators can be voted out of office if they do not represent the views of the majority of citizens. Thus as legislators seek consensus between competing forces, the laws they enact reflect changing social values. Aside from Nebraska, which has only one chamber, all states and the federal government have two legislative bodies that have the authority to enact laws. Legislative bills arise in either house of the state legislature or federal congress, sponsored by a private member or group of members. Bills are first referred to the appropriate committee. At scheduled hearings, this committee will solicit the viewpoints of interested citizens or groups. Amendments may be made to the bill before it gets out of committee or afterwards when it is read before the house. Eventually the house votes on the bill. If passed, the proposed legislation is referred to the equivalent committee in the second chamber. There it is discussed and amended if necessary. If the bill does not "die" in committee, it is reported to the second chamber for debate and possible amendment. If the bill passes the second chamber in amended form, the first chamber must approve the amendments. If not, the bill runs the risk of dying once again. If the amendments are approved, both houses sign the bill and refer it to the president or governor. The senior executive may sign the bill, fail to sign it, or veto it. If the executive refuses to sign, it may yet take effect after 10 days. If a piece of legislation successfully negotiates these hurdles, the two houses must next determine how, and to what extent, they will fund its implementation. They may do so by voting appropriations. Appropriation bills commonly originate in the state and federal house of representatives and are reviewed in the senates. Often, one bill will combine all the funds required by different agencies to implement several legislative entities.

In interpreting legislation, courts and governmental agencies seek to define legislative intent. Thus, they try to remain within the framework of existing law, for only the legislature is empowered to enact law. Courts and agencies may restrict their interpretations to the law's literal meaning or extend it in accordance with their understanding of the law's broader social purpose (i.e., the public good the legislation was intended to advance). I have already alluded to the ever-contentious question of how much latitude the courts should be allowed in interpreting legislation.

D. THE COURT SYSTEM

1. Federal Courts

Federal district courts are trial courts that hear cases arising under federal law such as tax evasion, civil rights infringements, claims for entitlements under federal law, crimes perpetrated on federal property, the transportation of illicit drugs, and interstate disputes in which the amount involved exceeds $10,000. There are 11 regional *federal circuit courts* that hear cases on appeal from the federal district courts.

The *United States Supreme Court* is the court of last resort. Its function is to interpret the Constitution with regard to appeals against the holdings of federal or state appellate courts. Appellants may petition the Court to issue writ of certiorari (i.e., an order to a lower court to certify a case record and send it up for a hearing); but the Court has the discretion to grant or deny any petition. As a rule, the Supreme Court chooses to hear cases arising from social policy disputes that involve substantive constitutional questions. For example, in a series of cases (e.g., *Roe v. Wade* 1973; *Planned Parenthood of Central Missouri v. Danforth* 1976; *Bellotti v. Baird* 1976; *H.L. v. Matheson* 1981), the Court has sought to balance the legitimate desire of the State to regulate abortion against the right of its citizens to privacy, the right and competence of minors to make decisions about their own health, and the right of parents to rear their families without interference by the State.

2. State Courts

In different states, the functions of the *courts of inferior jurisdiction* may be assumed by a *magistrate's court,* a *municipal court,* a *traffic court,* or a *justice of the peace.* These courts deal with minor cases such as speeding, ordinance violations, and small claims disputes.

Criminal cases involving misdemeanors are usually heard in *district court* or *county court.* Felonies, appeals from district courts, injunctions, and restraining orders are commonly heard in a venue known variously as a *superior, trial,* or *circuit court,* or a *court of common pleas.* The superior court is a court of record (i.e., a court that keeps transcripts of hearings). Some states interpose an intermediate appellate court between the trial court and the state supreme court.

The *family court* is a court of special jurisdiction. It may also be known as a *domestic relations court* or *juvenile court.* The family court is a court of record that disposes of cases involving marital separation, divorce, child abuse and neglect, and offenses committed by minors. The *probate* or *chancery court* is a court of record and special jurisdiction dealing with wills, trusts, estates, guardianship, and conservancy.

The *state supreme court* is the state's court of last resort. In some states, a citizen has the right of appeal to the state supreme court; in others, the state supreme court has discretion over which suits it will hear. Within the state system, appeals are directed from superior court (in some states via an intermediate appellate court) to the state supreme court. From there, appeals may be directed by writ of habeas corpus to the U.S. district court or by writ of certiorari or via direct appeal to the U.S. Supreme Court.

E. JUDICIAL PROCEEDINGS

The four types of judicial proceedings are *criminal, quasicriminal, civil,* and *administrative.* Each of these will be described in turn.

1. Criminal Proceedings

Criminal prosecutions involve offenses punishable by execution, imprisonment, or fine. In criminal actions, the prosecution must prove its case against the accused "beyond a reasonable doubt" (see section F3, "Standards of Proof"). The accused must be afforded full due process—in other words, the right to be informed of the offense for which he or she is charged; a speedy public trial with judge, jury, and counsel; the right to present witnesses on his or her own behalf; and the right to confront and cross-examine the other side's witnesses. After the detention and booking of the accused, the State must show at an initial hearing that it has sufficient reason ("probable cause") to pursue the case further. Misdemeanor charges may be tried forthwith. Those charged with felonies are further detained, released on bail, or released on their own recognizance.

The attorney general's department is empowered to decide whether there is sufficient evidence to pursue a case, to determine the grade of offense with which the accused will be charged, and to plea bargain with the defendant. The State's attorney, who is employed by the office of the district attorney or attorney general, acts as the prosecutor in criminal cases. The accused is represented by a defense attorney who may be privately retained, appointed by the court, or provided by the public defender's office. The clerk of the court collates documents for the judge and schedules the docket of cases. Probation officers prepare presentence reports. Child welfare caseworkers prepare diagnostic or periodic review reports for the family court.

At various points, defense counsel will lodge *motions*, for example, to discover the prosecution's case or to suppress certain elements of the case. Next, at a *prima facie hearing* (Latin for "on the face of it") before a magistrate or judge or at an *indictment* before a *grand jury*, the prosecution will attempt to substantiate that it has sufficient evidence against the accused to proceed with the case.

At the next hearing, the *arraignment*, the accused pleads "guilty," "not guilty," "nolo contendere," or "not guilty by reason of insanity." Guilty pleas are usually lodged after plea bargaining, as a result of which the accused agrees to plead guilty to a lesser charge than that for which he or she had originally been indicted. Defendants who plead guilty may be dealt with at arraignment. Those who plead not guilty or not guilty by reason of insanity proceed to trial.

A *jury trial* begins with the *empaneling of the jury.* In many states, 12-person juries are required for felony cases; however, 6-member juries are increasingly common. Next, in *opening statements,* the prosecution and defense outline their sides of the case. The State presents the evidence against the accused through material exhibits and the direct examination of witnesses. The defense may challenge the materiality of the evidence presented, object to the *direct examination* of the prosecuting counsel, and *cross-examine* the State's witnesses. The defense then presents its case through exhibits, documents, and witnesses. Any of these may be challenged, objected to, or cross-examined by the prosecution. Throughout the trial the judge keeps order and rules on points of procedure, thus ensuring that the rules of evidence are followed.

When the evidence has been presented, the defense may lodge a *motion for acquittal*. If this motion is unsuccessful, each side *summates its case,* the judge *instructs the jury* as to the law, and the *jury retires* to find the facts of the case and to consider their verdict (which must usually be unanimous). "Finding the facts" refers to the task of determining which of the evidence is true. If the jury cannot agree, a new trial is held. If the accused is found not guilty, he or she is discharged.

If the verdict is guilty, a *dispositional hearing* is scheduled for sentencing. In determining the appropriate disposition or sentence for the guilty party, the judge will take into account all aspects of the case (e.g., the defendant's past record, presentence reports from probation officers, and reports from mental health clinicians). Sentencing usually involves a fine, probation, or imprisonment.

The state is not permitted to appeal an acquittal. The defendant, however, may *appeal a verdict or sentence* on the grounds of fact (e.g., insufficient evidence) or legal error (e.g., improperly obtained evidence). Infrequently, the defendant will lodge a *writ of habeas corpus* asserting that his or her detention is illegal because the trial was improper. The defendant may be released before serving the full sentence if, at a subsequent *dispositional review,* his or her behavior is considered to have been good or if other mitigating circumstances (e.g., advanced age) are held to apply.

2. Quasicriminal Proceedings

Juvenile delinquency hearings differ from criminal proceedings in that diversion, reformation, and treatment are emphasized more than punishment and retribution. The laws of arrest apply to juveniles: *Miranda* warnings must be given to the juvenile before a confession is sought, and probable cause must be established before a magistrate if the accused is to be detained. At the *probable cause hearing,* juvenile probation staff present evidence concerning the alleged offense, the juvenile's background and past history, the family's capacity to supervise the juvenile, and the juvenile's attitude toward the offense. After the probable cause hearing, the juvenile may be *released* or *diverted* (e.g., for mental health treatment), or *petitions* may be filed for *adjudication*. In cases involving particularly heinous offenses or incorrigibility, a petition may be filed for *transfer* ("waiver") to adult court.

If the case is not waived to adult court, it proceeds to an *adjudicatory hearing*, at which a judge decides whether the alleged act or acts were committed. The prosecution and the defense present evidence and cross-examine witnesses. After *In re Gault* (1969), the accused must be provided with extensive due process safeguards short of jury trial and a standard of proof "beyond a reasonable doubt." At the dispositional hearing, the judge has a wide range of rehabilitative options, such as dismissal, fine, probation, community service, hospitalization, residential placement, or confinement in a correctional facility. Juvenile court decisions may be reviewed at the discretion of appellate courts.

3. Civil Court Proceedings

Civil court proceedings resolve disputes between private citizens, for example, contests concerning child custody or liability for damages on the grounds of negligence. Because loss of liberty is not at stake, the standard of proof is usually "a preponderance of the evidence," although a "clear and convincing" standard is now required in hearings concerning the termination of parental rights (see section on "Standards of Proof").

The case begins with legal maneuvering. The plaintiff files a *complaint,* to which the defendant gives a formal, written *answer.* Both sides may pose *interrogatories* (lists of questions) for the other side to answer. The defendant may make a *motion to dismiss* the case, and either side may make a *motion to discover* the extent of the other side's case. Discovery is pursued through a review of documents and the deposition of witnesses.

At this point, many cases are settled. Indeed, some jurisdictions require a *pretrial conference* to promote settlement. If the case goes to trial, a jury will be *empaneled* or the case will be tried before a judge without a jury. The presentation of evidence and witnesses is similar to that in criminal proceedings. The plaintiff leads off. The defendant *moves for a directed verdict* (i.e., moves for the judge to declare that the defendant has no case to answer). If the directed verdict is disallowed, the defense presents *evidence in rebuttal*. Further *motions for directed verdicts* are presented. If these fail, the judge instructs the jury and the jury retires to find the facts and reach a *decision*. If it is not a jury trial, the judge retires to do so.

4. Administrative Hearings

The administrative proceeding most likely to involve child mental health professionals is the *due process hearing* conducted by state educational authorities. These hearings are mandated (by Public Law 94-142) whenever the parents of an educationally handicapped child are aggrieved by the identification, evaluation, placement, or education of the child. Parties to the hearing have the right to be represented by counsel, to present expert witnesses, and to cross-examine adverse witnesses. The proceedings are presided over by a specially appointed hearings officer (usually a judge or attorney). In general, the procedures followed in administrative hearings are similar to those in civil trials.

F. ADJUDICATION

This section deals with the rules of evidence, types of witnesses, standards of proof, and judicial reasoning involved in the American legal system.

1. The Rules of Evidence

Evidence refers to factual proofs concerning an issue at stake, presented during a trial for the purpose of convincing a judge or jury. Evidence is presented through witnesses, documents, or objects. It may be *direct* (e.g., through the testimony of an eyewitness) or *circumstantial* (i.e., inferred from a circumstance or chain of circumstances). The jury must decide whether the admissible evidence is *probative,* that is, whether it establishes the truth of an asserted fact. It is the judge's task to rule on whether particular evidence is material, competent, or relevant to the issue at stake and whether it has been legally obtained. *Material evidence* bears on the substantive legal issues in the case. *Competent evidence* is evidence that tends to establish the fact at issue directly—not as a result of speculation. *Relevant evidence* is material evidence tending to show that the specific fact at issue is likely to be true. *Hearsay evidence* is generally excluded because its veracity cannot be tested. Admissions made by a party to an action may be allowed as evidence, even admissions inferred by silence. Excited utterances overheard in the emotional aftermath of an incident (e.g., a rape) may be admissible. Public records (e.g., a register of birth) are generally exempt from the hearsay rule because they are regarded as reliable.

2. Types of Witnesses

It is the task of the judge or jury to determine whether a witness's testimony does or does not bear on the truth of the factual issues at stake (i.e., whether the witness is credible and material). Lay witnesses are limited to giving testimony concerning what they have seen, heard, or experienced first hand, and they must refrain from testifying about speculation, opinion, or hearsay.

Expert witnesses are called on to give evidence concerning matters that require knowledge or skill beyond that of laypersons. The expert must be qualified; in other words, he or she must be accredited by the court as having the expertise to speak to the issue at stake (e.g., the alleged negligence of a physician, the mental health of a defendant, or the quality of construction of a bridge). After accreditation, the expert may be asked to describe how he or she analyzed the issue at stake and what conclusion was reached, "with a reasonable degree of (medical, clinical, scientific) certainty." The judge must decide whether expert testimony is required, whether aspiring experts are qualified, and whether their testimony is material and relevant. The jury decides whether experts are credible and whether their testimony is probative.

3. Standards of Proof

The courts apply three different standards of proof in reaching a verdict: *proof beyond a reasonable doubt, proof by clear and convincing evidence,* and *proof by a preponderance of the evidence.* The most exacting standard, "beyond a reasonable doubt," applies to criminal proceedings. Based on the evidence presented, the State must convince the court that there can be no reasonable doubt that the accused is guilty as charged. The stringency of this standard is a protection against depriving the innocent of their liberty, an error considered more serious than allowing the guilty to go free. The "clear and convincing" standard applies to certain civil proceedings. It refers to proof sufficient to convince a prudent person, but not beyond reasonable doubt. The termination of parental rights, for example, requires a clear and convincing level of evidentiary proof (*Santosky v. Kramer* 1982). Civil cases (e.g., small claims disputes, child custody litigations, and civil liability suits) require the third level of proof: "a preponderance of the evidence." When following this doctrine, the judge or jury make their decision according to which side of a dispute carries the greater probative weight.

A fourth standard, "probable cause," applies to arrests, searches, seizures, and the warranting of such procedures. Before they enter premises to get evidence and before they search or arrest suspects, the police must show, or be prepared to show, that they have sufficient reason to suspect wrongdoing. "Probable cause" relates to circumstances that would lead a reasonably prudent person to believe that another person is committing or has committed a crime, even though there may be some room for doubt. As a rough guide, the "beyond a reasonable doubt," "clear and convincing," "preponderance," and "probable cause" standards refer, respectively, to 90%, 75%, 51%, and 25% levels of certainty.

4. Judicial Reasoning

A judge is a public officer appointed to preside over a court of law. In a jury trial, the judge keeps order and rules on all points of law or discretion; for example, the judge decides whether there is sufficient evidence to allow a trial to proceed, whether an expert witness is properly qualified, or whether a particular piece of evidence is admissible. If the case is tried without a jury, as in family court, the judge must also find the facts; in other words, he or she must sift the evidence to decide what has been proven. Thus, when two witnesses give differing testimony on a matter at issue, the judge must decide who is the more credible. In a jury trial, the jurors must find the facts. Before they do so, however, the judge may summarize the evidence and instruct them on the points of law that are at issue in the case. For example, if a plea of "not guilty by reason of insanity" has been entered, the judge will inform the jury concerning the legal test for insanity in that jurisdiction.

Judicial reasoning pivots around the legal issues at stake. The judge progressively collates, sifts, analyzes, and interprets documents and evidence to find the facts in light of these legal issues. The issues are generally determined early, but may be modified as the case proceeds by amendments to the pleadings or by the evidence presented at the trial. From a judge's vantage point, the serial steps involved in a case are as follows:

- Review of the file to ascertain the urgency and complexity of the case.
- Scheduling of events in accordance with the age of the case, its urgency and type (e.g., criminal or divorce), the need for discovery, the likelihood of pretrial motions, and the estimated duration of the trial.
- Disposition of preliminary matters such as the scope of discovery and the pretrial motions. The judge tries to ensure that the case is ready for final disposition promptly, affording counsel reasonable opportunity to be heard and to prepare their case for trial.
- Trial of the case, during which the judge gives both sides full opportunity to present evidence and to be heard on objections and

provides prompt, unbiased rulings based on law and justice.

- The decision, which may be provided orally at the end of a non-jury trial in uncomplicated cases or, in other circumstances, taken under advisement until a written decision is provided at a later date. Counsel may be allowed to submit written briefs to assist the judge in making the final decision. In a jury trial, the judge gives instructions on the law to the jury, who are charged with finding the facts and reaching a verdict.
- Postdecision events that may arise if a party petitions to reopen the case or to have the court reconsider its decision.

During these steps, a judge reads the file; collates the salient information; abstracts the central issues; considers the law relevant to the issues; receives the evidence during the hearing and sifts it for the facts that are relevant to the issues at stake; considers whether the facts are complete or adequate for the purposes of making a decision; determines the law that is applicable by reviewing case law precedents in accordance with the issues and facts of the case; weighs the facts in light of the law, justice, and common sense; and finally reaches a decision, citing the facts and the law that apply to the case.

To pursue these steps consistently, judges must embody certain attitudinal qualities. Both before and during the hearing, judges must tolerate a degree of uncertainty, avoid rushing to premature decisions, and continually review the facts in the light of new evidence. When writing the decision, judges avoid mere recitation of evidence. Instead, they find the credible facts and cite the evidence on which they are based, while attempting to understand and control personal bias and to consider the case from the standpoint of each party. Finally, judges should be aware that prompt judgments are important, for the law's delay can be more harmful than a wrong decision.

5. Case Law and Precedent

Case law is an assemblage of precedents. The purpose of the legal doctrine of precedent is to ensure that similar disputes are treated similarly. Counsel may contend that a ruling in a case from a different jurisdiction should be persuasive, but the judge must decide whether the past case is sufficiently similar to the present one to have any priority. In making this determination, a judge will examine which facts in the preceding case were taken into account in reaching that judgment and whether the court's reason for reaching the decision in the previous case is relevant to judging the present case. Legal precedents are not absolutely binding; they can be overruled if changes in public attitudes and policy dictate doing so. In an appellate case, the judicial opinion may be arranged in the following sections: the parties to the dispute; the point of law at issue; the holding of the lower court; the facts of the case; the legal issue in question in the appeal; the holding of the appellate court (with reasons and precedents); the dissenting opinion, if any; and the likely effect of the current decision on future cases. As the forensic clinician becomes more familiar with importance of legal precedents, he or she will read landmark cases and important new holdings with interest and benefit.

G. LEGAL ADVOCACY

The terms "lawyer," "counsel," and "attorney" are synonymous. They refer to a person who is licensed to practice law, that is, a person authorized to offer legal advice and to prosecute or defend cases in courts of law. A lawyer has graduated from a recognized law school and been admitted by examination to the bar of the state in which he or she practices. Lawyers are employed privately, by government, and by business corporations and labor unions. Private practitioners may be generalists or specialists in such fields as criminal, family, tort, tax, corporation, real estate, probate, or labor law. Mental health clinicians are most likely to encounter attorneys who practice privately in the fields of criminal, family, juvenile, and tort law; trial lawyers employed by the district attorney's or public defender's office; and state agency attorneys specializing in family, child welfare, or mental health law.

When consulted by a client, an attorney first ascertains the nature of the dispute for which the client seeks help. Is it a legal matter? Is it worth pursuing further? Are there avenues for resolution or redress that would be preferable to litigation? If the matter were to be litigated, could the client sustain the economic, emotional, and social costs of the action?

In many cases, legal research is required. When briefing an opinion on a case, the attorney hunts for case precedents, statutes, regulations, or ordinances that bear on the issue at stake in order to predict judicial opinion. The attorney will often proffer to the court a legal brief that analyzes the law pertinent to the case. By doing so, he or she hopes to persuade the judge to rule in a particular way.

Legal briefs sometimes include information acquired through medical, psychological, or sociological research. A mental health professional may be asked by the attorney to submit an affidavit—a document in which the affiant expert attests to a fact or facts relevant to a case (e.g., the psychopathology of sexually abused children). Affidavits often require substantiation by testimony in court.

The sequence of events in judicial proceedings has already been described. Attorneys represent their clients throughout the legal process. Actually, most cases never come to trial, but are dismissed, dealt with at arraignment, settled out of court, or allowed to die of neglect. Wise attorneys will sometimes persuade their clients to accept an early resolution (e.g., by plea bargaining or settling out of court) instead of undergoing the expense, uncertainty, and stress of protracted litigation.

The attorney's primary obligation is to represent the client in the most effective manner, for the adversary system works best when each side advocates its own case skillfully and vigorously tests the merit of the other side's case. The direct examination of an effective expert witness can be very persuasive. Ideally, the direct examination should be followed by a well-informed cross-examination by opposing counsel.

Scientists and clinicians operate in a world of probabilities. Many clinical ideas, although admittedly hypothetical in nature, are grist for the mill of clinical reasoning. Incompletely substantiated speculations, however, do not reach the level of certitude required by the courts. Expert witnesses who refer to such concepts should not be surprised if they are challenged by opposing counsel on these grounds.

No case is perfect. Complex arguments always contain flaws that await exploitation by the other side. Indeed, astute attorneys may bring out such weaknesses during the direct examination of expert witnesses to deflate the sails of the cross-examiner. Generally, however, counsel do not present a balanced case. Instead, as polemicists, they present the best argument possible for their client and attack the opposition's case whenever the opportunity presents. Failure to appreciate this fundamental difference between clinical work, scientific research, and the law leads to much friction between the mental health and legal professions.

H. SUMMARY

Clinicians who enter the forensic arena should understand the nature and purposes of the law and the way in which it differs from science and clinical work. Scientists seek to approximate the truth with regard to the relationship between things and events. Clinicians aim to diagnose and treat sick or troubled individuals and families. The law proposes to settle disputes impartially, justly, and mercifully. It does so in a formalized tug-of-war known as the adversary system, a system that requires each side to test the validity of its opponent's case, thereby exposing the facts for the court to ponder.

American law is derived from the federal Constitution, particularly the First, Fourth, Fifth, Sixth, Eighth, and Fourteenth Amendments. It also is derived from statutes and ordinances enacted by Congress, state legislatures, and town councils. The common law is a collection of customs and precedents inherited from English law. Case law refers to the legal reasoning and holdings of federal and state appellate courts. The holdings of state appellate courts are binding over courts of inferior jurisdiction in the same state, whereas the holdings of federal appellate courts have precedent over state courts. There are three levels in the federal court system: district courts, courts of appeal, and the U.S. Supreme Court (the court of last resort). The hierarchy in state courts involves courts of inferior jurisdiction, district courts, family courts, probate courts, superior courts, and supreme (appellate) courts.

Different courts try different kinds of cases: criminal, juvenile, civil, and administrative. Cases are tried during formalized proceedings that culminate in a verdict or decision. Courts are bound by rules of evidence, and different standards of proof are required in different kinds of cases. In contrast to a clinical diagnosis, which requires a balanced exposition of a patient's strengths and weaknesses, legal arguments are polemic. Each lawyer attempts to put forward the strongest support for his or her client and to challenge the validity of the other side's case. Failure to appreciate the principle and purpose of the adversary system confuses clinicians who are unfamiliar with the courts.

I. SELECTED READINGS

Two books provide helpful introductions to the law for the mental health clinician without legal training: *Law for the Layman* (Coughlin 1975) and *The Law and the Practice of Human Services* (Woody 1984). The former is a general introduction; the latter is written specially for mental health and human services professionals. As the title implies, *Law and Social Work Practice* (Albert 1986) contains detailed references to legislation, administration, and child welfare. It is particularly relevant to the needs of social workers. Slovenko's (1973) *Psychiatry and Law* contains an excellent chapter on evidence, the adversary system, the credibility of testimony, and privileged communication. *Psychological Evaluations for the Courts* (Melton et al. 1987) has informative chapters on paradigm differences between the legal and the mental health professions, the definition of expertise, and an overview of the sources of law, the courts, and the adjudicative process. *Law and Psychiatry* (Moore 1984) provides an original analysis of the difference between the legal and the psychodynamic views of insanity. Moore has suggested that both

legal and mental health professionals could benefit from a more philosophical perspective on their fields.

J. TABLE OF CASES

American Academy of Pediatrics v Heckler, 561 F Supp 395 [DDC (1983)]
Bellotti v Baird, 428 US 132 (1976)
Brown v Topeka Board of Education, 347 US 483 (1954)
In re Gault, 387 US 1 (1967)
Griswold v Connecticut, 381 US 479 (1965)
H.L. v Matheson, 450 US 398 (1981)
Hazelwood School District v Kuhlmeier, 56 USLW 4079 (1988)
Kent v US, 383 US 541 (1966)
Morales v Turman, 383 F Supp 53 (ED Tex 1971)
Planned Parenthood of Central Missouri v Danforth, 428 US 52 (1976)
Roe v Wade, 410 US 113 (1973)
Santosky v Kramer, 455 US 745 (1982)
Tinker v Des Moines Independent School District, 393 US 503 (1969)
In re TLO, 94 NJ 331, 463 A2d 934, cert granted, 52 USLW 3413 (Nov 29,
    1983)

K. REFERENCES

Albert R: Law and Social Work Practice. New York, Springer, 1986
Coughlin GG: Law for the Layman. New York, Harper & Row, 1975
Faust D, Ziskin J: The expert witness in psychology and psychiatry. Science
    241:31–35, 1988
Melton GB, Petrila J, Poythress NG, et al: Psychological Evaluations for the
    Courts: A Handbook for Mental Health Professionals and Lawyers. New
    York, Guilford, 1987
Moore MS: Law and Psychiatry. Rethinking the Relationship. New York,
    Cambridge, 1984
Morse S: Crazy behavior, morals and science: an analysis of mental health
    laws. Southern California Law Review 51:600–619, 1978
Slobogin C: The role of mental health professionals in the clinical process:
    the case for informed speculation. Virginia Law Review 66:452–495,
    1980

Slovenko R: Psychiatry and Law. Boston, MA, Little Brown, 1973
Woody RH (ed): The Law and the Practice of Human Services. San Francisco,
    CA, Jossey-Bass, 1984

CHAPTER TEN

Legal Issues Commonly Requiring Mental Health Consultation

Barry Nurcombe, M.D.

C linicians are most likely to be involved in legal matters in the following circumstances: child custody disputes, allegations of child neglect or maltreatment, the termination of parental rights, civil liability suits, clinical malpractice, the evaluation of juvenile offenders, and cases requiring an understanding of mental health law. To evaluate cases of this type and give expert testimony if called on, clinicians should be aware of the principles of constitutional, statutory, and case law that guide legal reasoning in these matters. Only in that way will their reports and testimony elucidate the legal questions that attorneys must address and the courts must cogitate. Furthermore, the clinician should be aware of empirical research in areas such as the psychological effects of divorce, child maltreatment, traumatic stress, and the prediction of dangerousness in offenders and psychiatric patients. A full exposition of legal principles and scientific research is beyond the scope of an introductory text. This chapter presents only the basic principles.

A. CHILD CUSTODY DISPUTES

1. Legal Doctrines

The evolution of legal reasoning with regard to child custody illustrates the flux that characterizes family law, a flux that reflects changing community standards concerning the status of women, the permanence of marriage, the legitimate grounds for divorce, and the rights of children.

a. Maternal preference

During the nineteenth century and the first half of the twentieth century, mothers were regarded as the proper custodians after divorce. This, the "tender years" doctrine, was toppled in New York (*State ex. rel. Watts v. Watts* 1973) Louisiana (*Ex parte Devine* 1981) and Utah (*Pusey v. Pusey* 1986) on the grounds that discrimination against fathers violated their Fourteenth Amendment equal protection rights. By 1990, only one state (Tennessee) deferred to parental sex, and only then if the child was under 30 months of age. One unanticipated result of the displacement of maternal preference has been the encouragement of custody litigation.

b. Best interests of the child

In recent years, the concept of the child's best interests has prevailed. Many states have codified the elements of this doctrine in accordance with the Uniform Marriage and Divorce Act (1970) that was promulgated by the American Bar Association, as follows:

The court shall determine custody in accordance with the best interests of the child. The court shall consider all relevant factors, including

1. The wishes of the child's parent or parents as to his custody
2. The wishes of the child as to his custodian

3. The interaction and interrelationship of the child with his parent, his sibling, and any other person who may significantly affect the child's best interests
4. The child's adjustment to his home, school, and community
5. The mental and physical health of all individuals involved

The relevant section (722.33) of the Michigan Child Custody Act (1970) adds to the above criteria considerations such as the love, affection, and other emotional ties between the competing parties and the child; the parties' relative capacity to give the child love, affection, guidance, education, food, and medical or remedial care; the desirability of maintaining continuity of care; the moral fitness of the competing parties; and their mental and physical health. Judges have broad discretion in applying these criteria. Clinicians should be aware of the statutory criteria or case precedents that prevail in the local state, and address them in the forensic evaluation (see Chapter 11).

c. Continuity of care

In some states, preference is given to the parent who, at the time of the custody hearing, is the child's primary caretaker with regard to meals, bedtime, grooming, clothing, medical care, social activities, discipline, education, religion, and basic skills. In reality, if the mother was nominated as custodian in the initial court order, it may be difficult for the father to prevail in the face of the continuity-of-care argument, particularly if there is any residual "tender years" bias on the judge's part.

2. Types of Custody

a. Single parent custody

In this, the commonest form of custody, the custodial parent makes all decisions concerning the child's care, control, education, health, and religion. The noncustodial parent may or may not be awarded visitation.

b. Joint parental custody

Joint custody entails legal custody (the authority to make decisions concerning the child's life) and physical custody (the child's primary domicile). Physical custody may or may not be alternated between the parents. Sometimes joint legal custody is awarded together with sole physical custody. The states vary from presuming joint custody to be preferable (e.g., Louisiana) to presuming it is inimical to the best interests of the child (e.g., Vermont).

3. Controversial Issues

a. Moral unfitness

Claims of moral unfitness are less frequent than heretofore because divorce today usually is on a "no fault" basis. To be awarded custody or to regain it, a parent must prove that the other parent's irregular life-style directly affects the child. For example, parental drug taking or sexual activity in the presence of the child is likely to debar custody (e.g., as in *Harrison v. Harrison* [1978]).

b. Parental mental illness or impairment

Theoretically, parental mental illness (e.g., psychosis, personality disorder, drug abuse, or mental retardation) should be taken into account only insofar as it affects child-rearing. In practice, mental disorder often weighs heavily against the afflicted parent (e.g., *In re Bachelor* 1973).

c. Child's religion or race

Because of the First Amendment right to freedom of religion, the courts are reluctant to base a custody award primarily on religion or race, although it may be considered as one of a number of factors (*Palmore v. Sidoti* 1984).

d. Child's preference

The child's preference, if not unreasonable, may be considered as one of a number of factors influencing the determination of custody (e.g., *Witmayer v. Witmayer* 1983). In some jurisdictions (e.g., Minnesota and New Jersey), the child's wishes must be ascertained. In practice, the wishes of an adolescent are difficult to override, unless they are patently unreasonable or inappropriate.

e. Siblings

Recognizing the desirability of maintaining residual family ties, the courts are reluctant to split siblings unless it can be shown that such separation would be in their best interests (e.g., *Johnson v. Lundell* 1958).

f. Substantial change of circumstances

To modify an existing custody or visitation award, for example to regain custody, a noncustodial parent must establish that the original circumstances have changed and that the change has favorably or unfavorably affected (or would affect) the child's welfare (e.g., *Christian v. Randall* 1973).

g. Relocation of the custodial parent

Although many custody awards enjoin parents from leaving the home state, such clauses are probably unenforceable (*Bloss v. Bloss* 1985). Some courts require a hearing before such a move, but most do not (e.g., *McIntyre v. McIntyre* 1984).

h. Allegations of sexual abuse

Accusations of sexual abuse have become more frequent during custody disputes or afterwards, when visitation is at issue. Such claims represent a potent method of barring the noncustodial parent from access to the child. These allegations vary from genuine and well-founded (or sincere but erroneous) to false and malicious. The characteristics of erroneous, false, deluded, and true accusations are described in Chapter 11.

i. Rights of grandparents

In common law, grandparents had no legal right to access to their grandchildren. However, a number of judgments have allowed grandparents to have contact when it was deemed to be in the child's best interests (e.g., *Looper v. McManus* 1978). Furthermore, if a child has lived with grandparents for a substantial time, the court may find it to be in the child's best interests to remain with them (e.g., *Wrecsis v. Broughton* 1981).

j. Child snatching

The kidnapping of children by noncustodial parents can have serious psychological effects (e.g., Senior et al. 1983). In 1968, the Uniform Child Custody Jurisdiction Act provided that the state issuing the original custody award should retain jurisdiction; however, not all states adopted this act. In 1980, Congress passed the Parental Kidnapping Prevention Act, which enjoined all states from modifying custody determinations made in other states. The Federal Bureau of Investigation was empowered to arrest offenders and turn them over to the state authorities pending extradition. All states but one have enacted laws that enable parental kidnappers to be tried as felons. Moreover, child victims of parental kidnapping have the option of bringing civil suit against offenders on the grounds of psychological injury.

k. Lesbian parents

Despite contrary psychological evidence (see the review by Hutchens and Kirkpatrick 1985), homosexuals are popularly thought to be psychologically unstable, pedophilic, or likely to raise children who will assume irregular or immoral life-styles.

Undoubtedly, some judges are biased against homosexuals. However, the modern trend is to assess each case in accordance with the child's best interests. In several decisions (e.g., *Bezio v. Patenaude* 1980; *DiStefano v. DiStefano* 1978) the key question was whether the parent's personal life intruded adversely on child-rearing.

4. Effects of Divorce on Children

The major longitudinal studies in this field are the California study (Kelly and Wallerstein 1976; Wallerstein 1983; Wallerstein and Blakeslee 1989; Wallerstein and Kelly 1975, 1976, 1980a, 1980b), the Virginia study (Hetherington 1984, 1989; Hetherington and Clingempeel 1992; Hetherington et al. 1976, 1978, 1979, 1989), and studies by Billingham et al. (1989), Block et al. (1988), Buchanan et al. (1991), Furstenberg et al. (1987), Glenn and Kramer (1987), Guidibaldi (1988), and Johnston and Campbell (1988).

The California study concerned 131 children, 3–18 years of age, from 60 white, middle-class families who were followed for 5 years after marital separation. The families were recruited through an offer of counseling and were thus essentially a clinical sample. Attrition was low. No control group was observed. All assessments were clinical and relatively unstandardized.

At the time of separation, the rupture of the family was universally disturbing. Few divorces were mutual, few children experienced relief, many were unaware that separation was pending, and only a minority were given an adequate explanation for the breakup. In the first year, parents often became irritable, aggressive, depressed, or even suicidal; and external support was frequently unavailable because of the remoteness of extended families. Commonly, marked changes in family relationships ensued. Some noncustodial parents became more or less involved than before, yet most children experienced a need to maintain contact with the absent parent.

All children experienced fear, anger, guilt, helplessness, a sense of loss, and divided loyalties. Preschool children tended to regress and express fear of abandonment. Children 5–8 years of age grieved the loss, felt rejected, and fantasized about reconciliation. In about half the cases, school performance deteriorated. At 9–12 years, children characteristically exhibited anger, grief, and loneliness, split their parents into "good" and "bad" parties, and blamed the "bad" one. About half had problems with school performance. Adolescents became anxious and concerned for their own marital futures.

Five years after the separation, about one-third of the children were in good psychological health. Good outcome was associated with the following: a stabilized family life, a continuing relationship with both parents, the severance of a relationship with an abusive parent, and the reduction of friction between parents. About 40% of the children were still clinically disturbed. Poor outcome was associated with the following: feelings of having been rejected by either parent; lack of interest by the noncustodial parent; chronic depression, embitterment, or ill health in the custodial mother; and the continuation of friction between the parents.

Wallerstein (1983) hypothesized that the following six coping tasks must be completed in order for the emotional crisis to be resolved:

1. Acknowledging the marital disruption
2. Regaining a sense of direction and resuming customary activities
3. Dealing with feelings of loss and rejection
4. Forgiving the parents
5. Accepting the finality of divorce
6. Resolving fear of adult relationships

Ten years after the divorce, a significant number of the older group (now 19–29 years of age) had upsetting memories of or amnesia about the earlier trauma. Others had become troubled, underachieving adults. Some young women, who had appeared well-adjusted during adolescence, had become anxious concerning love, intimacy, commitment, and betrayal. Some young men pursued a "counterphobic" life-style involving transient sex. Fifteen years subsequently, it has become apparent that events during the third decade of life (e.g., psychotherapy or establishing a different relationship with the father) can have a significant impact on adjustment. Although boys had more apparent difficulties during the first 10 years, girls began to show more problems during early adulthood, as evidenced by multiple relationships, early marriage, and early divorce.

The Virginia study followed 72 white, middle-class children 4–5 years of age, along with a matched control group, for 6 years after divorce. Standardized assessments were used. There was considerable attrition in the sample. If the parents agreed about child-rearing and there was little conflict between them, frequent paternal contact was associated with better mother-child relationships. If conflict continued, or the father was emotionally immature, frequent paternal visitation was disruptive to the child. No other relationship outside the home had such potential for good or ill as that with the father. Sex differences were noted among the children's responses. Emotional disturbance tended to disappear among girls after 2 years (although it might reappear in adolescence). In contrast, many boys remained disturbed at 2 years, exhibiting oppositional, aggressive behavior. Boys appeared to be exposed to more stress, inconsistency, and rejection by mothers. Many families deteriorated economically after divorce, and the mother's working sometimes resulted in a chaotic life-style. If the mother remained hostile to the father, the boy's gender role identity might be disturbed.

At 6-year follow-up, when the children were 10 years of age, sample attrition dictated the addition of new subjects, 30 sons and 30 daughters in each of three groups: remarried mother-stepfather; nonremarried mother custody; and nondivorced. Mother-son relationships in the nonremarried families and parent-child relationships in the remarried families tended to be problematic. In the first 2 years after remarriage, mother-daughter relations were likely to deteriorate, whereas mother-son relations often stabilized. Stepfathers appeared to relate better to their stepsons than to their stepdaughters. Several adaptive clusters were defined among the children:

1. Insecure, aggressive, impulsive, and withdrawn
2. Self-sufficient, energetic, and popular, but manipulative and opportunistic
3. Warm, compassionate, and sharing (mostly girls)

In a recent, allied study, Hetherington and Clingempeel (1992) reported the results of research into the effect on children of parental remarriage. Cohorts of nondivorced, divorced, and re-married families were studied, at an average of 4, 17, and 26 months after remarriage. It was apparent that remarriage was par-ticularly disruptive, and that there was little improvement in the resulting disturbance during the first 2 years of follow-up. Ado-lescent daughters often became oppositional toward their stepfa-thers, who tended to withdraw from limit-setting and discipline. Adolescent daughters also often became oppositional toward their mothers. Nevertheless, authoritative parenting was associated with better outcome. The especially disruptive effect of parental remarriage on daughters and the failure of remarried families to readjust within 2 years represent the most challenging findings of this study.

The Johnston and Campbell (1988) study concerned a 4-year follow-up of 100 children of parents who were disputing custody. Seventy percent of the children were exposed to verbal and phys-ical abuse between their parents. Younger children tended to be-come inhibited and "frozen," particularly at times of transition from home to home. Older children often became embroiled in the parental struggle. Many children blamed themselves for the conflict. After 2 years, aggression, depression, and manipulative behavior were evident, especially among boys. Other children had learned, like chameleons, to "merge" with either parent. Four years after the parental separation, children in court-ordered joint custody arrangements were significantly more disturbed than those in single-parent custody. Mother-daughter relationships, particularly, had deteriorated in court-ordered shared custody ar-rangements. Many girls tended to develop seductive, manipula-tive relationships with their fathers and hostility toward their mothers. Court-ordered shared custody was regarded as deleterious. The Stanford study (Buchanan et al. 1991) also found that dual residence was harmful to adolescents who felt trapped between parents in conflict.

The National Survey of Children (Furstenberg et al. 1987) examined the long-term effect of divorce on several thousand children, comparing them with controls from intact families. As expected, children of divorced families were worse off in regard to school performance, problem behavior, and subjective distress. Younger children appeared to be more disturbed than older children, but the sex of the child had no effect. Another finding from this study was the widespread abandonment of children by their fathers.

In the National Study of Children in the Schools (Guidibaldi 1988), children from divorced families were compared with intact-family classroom controls 4 and 6 years after parental separation. Children from divorced families demonstrated poorer school performance, more psychological symptoms, and less popularity. Boys exhibited more adverse effects than girls. In national cross-sectional studies, Glenn and Kramer (1987) found an intergenerational effect in that the children of divorce are more likely as adults to be involved in divorce themselves. Women seem to be affected more than men, as adults, after having experienced parental divorce: they marry earlier but appear to be less committed to their marriages. Billingham et al. (1989) found that college women who had experienced parental divorce were likely to have more sexual partners yet to be less permissive in their attitudes toward sex.

Aside from the two major longitudinal studies, a large number of cross-sectional studies examined the relationship between children's psychological adjustment after divorce and different personal and environmental variables. Reviews of these studies have been provided by Wolchik and Karoly (1985) and Wallerstein (1991). The factors that appear to influence outcome adversely are postdivorce impoverishment, environmental instability, parental maladjustment, and continued parental conflict. These studues have not shown any clear effect based on age or sex.

B. CHILD MALTREATMENT

1. Legal Doctrines

a. Parens patriae

The State assumes its right to intervene in family life and appropriate the custody of neglected or maltreated children under the doctrine of *parens patriae*. This ancient principle of English chancery law originally empowered the King to step in to protect the interests of his mentally handicapped, mentally ill, or minor subjects. The U.S. Supreme Court upheld this doctrine in *Prince v. Massachusetts* (1944).

b. Best interests of the child

This doctrine, which emerged in the context of child custody disputes, has been held to override the Fourth Amendment rights of parents in cases of child maltreatment or neglect. In order to prevail in this matter, the State must show that the child is at serious risk of substantial physical or psychological harm.

2. Situations Giving Rise to Intervention

The situations likely to lead to State intervention usually involve physical abuse, neglect, abandonment, sexual abuse, emotional abuse, medical or educational neglect, or parental incapacity.

a. Physical abuse

All states mandate the reporting of suspected physical abuse; however, there is considerable variation in the definition of when legitimate discipline becomes illegal abuse. In most jurisdictions, "reasonable" force is accepted but no more than required to punish a child without substantial risk of physical or psychological injury. In *State v. Jones* (1886), chastisement based on "corrective authority" was contrasted with punishment based on "malice." Failure to follow mandatory reporting laws will expose clinicians to penalty of imprisonment or fine and to ultimate risk of civil action for negligence (e.g., *Landeros v. Flood* 1976).

b. Neglect and abandonment

Most actions are based on neglect or abandonment to a degree likely to be associated with the serious risk of imminent harm. In *Alsager v. District Court* (1975), Iowa's neglect statutes were held to be so vague that they denied parents due process. However, other decisions (e.g., *In re K.B.* 1981) have upheld the need for wide judicial discretion in these complex cases.

c. Sexual abuse

Without medical evidence, sexual abuse is difficult to substantiate, because it relies on the testimony of child witnesses, who are notoriously fragile. Children are most likely to be removed from sexually abusive environments when nonabusing parents are unable to protect them from further abuse.

d. Emotional abuse

Emotional abuse refers to the infliction of psychological harm on children as a result of persistent verbal and psychological rejection and depreciation. It is difficult to prove and is seldom the sole basis of a successful legal action.

e. Educational and medical neglect

Educational or medical neglect refers to failure to provide a child with proper schooling or medical care (e.g., by condoning truancy). It can also refer to the shunning of formal schooling or health care on the grounds of sincere religious conviction. In such cases, the courts will usually issue an emergency order for medical or mental health treatment but permit the child to remain in parental custody.

f. Parental incapacity

The parents most likely to be deemed incompetent to care for their children are those afflicted by alcohol or drug dependence, mental illness, or mental retardation. Expert opinion may be required to determine whether the parental problem is serious enough to place the child at substantial risk of physical or psychological harm. An opinion may also be required as to whether a child with exceptional medical, mental health, or educational needs could be adequately cared for by the parent in question.

3. Child Protection Hearings

Through their child protection systems, states aim to investigate claims of neglect or abandonment promptly, take legal action to protect endangered children, design and monitor plans for family reunification, or, if this is impossible, arrange permanent, stable placement. Because criminal proceedings require an exacting standard of proof, they are usually reserved for the most egregious offenses. Civil actions in family court are more expedient, more likely to lead to reunification, and better able to provide the court with a range of discretionary alternatives.

Civil proceedings open with an *emergency custody hearing* after the child has been removed from the home. The State subsequently files a petition for abuse or neglect. Sometimes a *civil protection order* will be sought to bar an abusive parent from the house. The State must subsequently prove its case at a *merits hearing*. At this hearing, the child will be represented by a guardian ad litem or an attorney, or both. Parents may be provided with an attorney if they are at risk of subsequent prosecution. Expert testimony may be required regarding the psychological health and prognosis of the child victim, the consistency of the pattern of signs and symptoms of maltreatment, and the competence of the parents or the likelihood they could be rendered competent by treatment. Dispositions available to the judge include dismissal, returning the child home for further diagnosis or treatment, or committing the child to state custody with reunification planning.

Although the state has assumed custody, parents retain residual rights (e.g., to consent to adoption or marriage) until and unless these rights are terminated.

The Federal Adoption Assistance and Child Welfare Act (1980) provides incentives to the states to encourage reunification or permanency planning and to avert foster care drift. The chief criteria for termination of parental rights are as follows: the failure of parents to rectify defects in their parenting competence; extreme parental incapacity; egregious abuse, neglect, or abandonment; and irretrievable breakdown in the parent-child relationship. Mental health clinicians may be called on to give expert testimony on these matters at proceedings that sever parental rights and free the child for adoption, guardianship, or long-term foster care.

4. Research Into the Effects of Sexual Abuse on Children

Mental health clinicians are most likely to be consulted as experts in child protection cases that involve alleged sexual abuse. The dimensions of sexual abuse include the sexes of the perpetrator and victim and the age discrepancy between them; the closeness of the kinship relationship between them; in the case of extrafamilial abuse, the familiarity of the perpetrator; the frequency of the abuse and the length of time over which it took place; the coerciveness of the abuse; and the nature of the sexual activity involved. Reviews of the immediate and long-term effects of intrafamilial and extrafamilial abuse were provided by Cicchetti and Carlson (1989), Finkelhor (1984), Haugaard and Reppucci (1988), Sgroi (1982), and Walker (1988).

The *immediate effects* of a single abuse experience vary from an adjustment reaction to acute posttraumatic stress disorder. Posttraumatic stress disorder is characterized by unbidden intrusive memories, trauma dreams, waking "flashbacks," reenactments, emotional numbing, amnesia, the avoidance of situations that remind the victim of the experience, hypervigilance, and emotional hyperarousal. It may evolve, in some cases, from an undifferentiated stress reaction.

The *intermediate effects* of repeated sexual abuse include

low self-esteem, guilt, a sense of powerlessness, depression, anger, sexually provocative behavior and play, sexual identity confusion, lack of trust, social withdrawal, aggressiveness, running away from home, antisocial behavior, self-injury, and suicide. Finkelhor and Browne (1985) postulated that the psychodynamics of incest involve a tetrad of characteristics: premature eroticization, a sense of betrayal, a sense of powerlessness, and stigmatization. The victims of sexual abuse are often entrapped in family relationships characterized by secrecy and threat, and they may be forced to accommodate to the abuse for long periods.

The *long-term consequences* that have been reported include sexual dysfunction, depression, suicide, substance abuse, chronically low self-esteem, prostitution, eating disorder, dissociative disorder, borderline personality disorder, the failure to protect offspring from being sexually abused, and, especially in males, the sexual victimization of others.

It is not clear whether the age or sex of the victim affects outcome; however, children with prior emotional disturbance may be especially vulnerable. Intrafamilial abuse, coercive abuse, and abuse of long duration appear to be particularly serious. A negative reaction by the parents to the child's disclosure of abuse, leading to out-of-home placement, may be especially adverse. Unusual situations that may be disturbing to children involve child prostitution, pornographic sex rings, and ritual abuse. In some cases, the distinction between these forms of abuse may be unclear (Nurcombe and Ünützer 1991).

C. CIVIL LIABILITY

1. Legal Doctrines

a. Definitions

A *tort* is an actionable civil wrong other than breach of contract arising when one party's act or omission causes damage to the person or property of another. An *unintentional tort* refers to damage arising from a negligent but not willful act or omission (e.g., when a careless driver injures a pedestrian). An *intentional tort* refers to an act or omission that the tortfeasor knew or ought to have known was wrong (e.g., when a careless or malicious physician damages the reputation of a patient by gossiping about him).

b. Elements of a negligent tort

To prove that a defendant was negligent and that compensation is warranted, the plaintiff must prove the following facts:

i. Duty. The defendant owed a *duty of care* to the plaintiff. In other words, the relationship between defendant and plaintiff was such that the defendant should have adhered to a standard of care in exercising his or her duty. For example, a dog owner should restrain his or her vicious pet, the pilot of an airplane should not drink alcohol when on duty, and an engineer should exercise due care when designing a bridge. The standard of care is established by the legislature (e.g., by enacting motor vehicle driving laws), by professional bodies (e.g., the American Psychiatric Association's statements on ethics), or by expert witnesses.

ii. Dereliction. The defendant was derelict in that duty. In other words, by act or omission, the defendant fell below the standard of care. For example, a dog owner allows a vicious dog to roam the streets; a drunken pilot flies an airplane; or a careless engineer designs a defective bridge.

iii. Damage. The dereliction of duty resulted in compensable harm to the plaintiff. Harm is defined as the invasion of a legally protected interest. It is not compensable unless the harm and the interest are judged to be sufficiently significant. For example, the negligent owner's dog bites and injures a child; the drunken pilot's airplane crashes and kills a passenger; or the engineer's bridge falls down and damages another person's house.

iv. Causation. In law, "causation" refers to a "but-for" situation in which the negligent act or omission was the necessary antecedent to the harm, either directly or through a foreseeable chain of events. For example, an unrestrained dog bites a child on the face, and the wound subsequently becomes infected and results in a disfiguring scar. The negligent dog owner may be liable for the medical expenses, pain and suffering associated with the original injury, and for the psychological damage of the disfigurement. The legal concept of causation is roughly synonymous with the clinical concepts of precipitation or aggravation.

c. Compensation

Injury to person or property can be compensated with money. Compensatory damages are awarded in an attempt to recoup the victim's losses in terms of pain and suffering, loss of earnings, medical expenses, and property damage. Punitive damages may be imposed if the judge wishes to make an example of a particularly outrageous wrongdoer.

d. Negligent infliction of emotional distress

Until the 1960s, the courts were inclined to disfavor suits brought on the grounds of psychological injury, largely for fear of opening the floodgates to a torrent of litigation. However, in *Batalla v. State of New York* (1961), a plaintiff recovered damages for mental injury after he had been left dangling from a defective ski lift. In *Tobin v. Grossman* (1964), the New York appellate court awarded damages to a mother who witnessed her child being struck by an automobile. In doing so, the court established two principles: 1) the plaintiff should be closely related to the primary victim; and 2) the plaintiff should also have been in the "zone of danger" (i.e., to have also been at risk of injury).

e. Preexisting condition

The law is said to take its victims as it finds them. If the victim had been psychologically disturbed before the injury in question, and the psychological disturbance became aggravated by the injury, compensation might be allowed.

f. Intentional torts

As previously defined, intentional torts involve deliberate or willful wrongdoing. The most common intentional torts are *assault* (putting a victim at reasonable fear of being injured), *battery* (unlawful harmful contact), and *slander* (false, damaging, written or broadcast communication). In medical malpractice, the most common intentional torts involve *breach of confidentiality* and *improper sexual contact*. In law, an intentional tort requires the substantiation of three elements:

i. A specific, volitional act. An act conducted under the influence of drugs or delirium is not actionable as an intentional tort.

ii. Intent. This refers to an intent to do something that could have damaging consequences. Intent is to be distinguished from motive. For example, a nurse may intend to lay hands on a patient but with the motive of getting the patient into the hospital for treatment.

iii. Injury. The intentional, volitional act must be the direct cause of compensable injury to the plaintiff or the proximate cause of a foreseeable chain of events that causes injury. For example, the nurse who intentionally laid hands on a patient (with the motive of getting him into the hospital) accidentally injures the patient.

2. Research

Most of the relevant research in this area has to do with the validity of the diagnosis of posttraumatic stress disorder in children, the natural history of childhood and adolescent posttraumatic stress disorder, and differences between posttraumatic stress disorder after single events (e.g., kidnapping, bushfire) and posttraumatic stress disorder after repeated events (e.g., sexual or physical abuse). Useful reviews have been provided by Pynoos and Eth (1984), McFarlane (1987), and Terr (1991).

D. MALPRACTICE

1. Definition

Malpractice is a form of tort that refers to an act or omission by a professional in the course of his or her duty that causes or aggravates an injury to a client or patient and that is the result of a failure to exercise due prudence, diligence, knowledge, or skill.

2. Legal Doctrines

a. Elements of malpractice

The plaintiff must substantiate the following four points:

- The professional owed a *duty of reasonable care* to the client. In other words, an implicit or explicit contract existed between them.
- Judged by the standard of the average prudent practitioner, the professional *breached the standard of care*. A professional is not liable for an error of judgment unless the error represented substandard care.
- The victim sustained *compensable injury* or harm. Harm may be physical or psychological.
- The breach of care was the *direct or proximate cause* of the injury.

An expert witness may be required to establish the standard of professional care, determine the nature and extent of the injury, and give an opinion concerning the connection between the breach of duty and the injury.

b. Fiduciary relationship

The clinician owes more than a duty of care to the patient. The clinician is obliged to act in the patient's best interests and to avoid double agentry by exploiting the patient for financial gain or sexual purposes.

c. Vicarious liability

Just as an employer may be liable for the negligence of an employee, a physician may be liable for the error of a nurse or resident.

d. Confidentiality and privilege

Confidentiality is the patient's right not to have private matters divulged. Privilege is the patient's right to bar his or her physician from divulging private matters in court. Exceptions to the rule of privilege apply when the patient waives it, when a person offers his or her mental health as evidence in litigation, when the person's mental health was examined as part of a case (e.g., in a child custody dispute), when an endangered third party must be protected, or when suspected child abuse must be reported.

e. Informed consent

The doctrine of informed consent is based on the individual's constitutional right to control his or her own body (*Schloendorff v. Society of New York Hospital* 1914). Patients cannot give informed consent unless they have sufficient information and adequate mental competence to make a rational decision—and unless they make their decision voluntarily. After *Canterbury v. Spence* (1971) and *Cobb v. Grant* (1971), some jurisdictions have switched the standard for consent from 1) *the information a responsible practitioner would disclose* to 2) *the information a reasonable patient would need in order to make a balanced decision.* It is recommended that practitioners discuss with individuals whom they propose to treat the nature of the diagnosis; the nature, purpose, risks, consequences, and likelihood of success of any proposed treatment; the nature, risks, consequences, and likelihood of success of alternative treatments; and the risks and consequences of providing no treatment. For minors, parental consent is required, except in emergencies. It is also desirable to seek the assent of children over 12 years of age.

f. Failure to protect endangered third parties

For full exposition of this, the Tarasoff doctrine (*Tarasoff v. Regents of the University of California* 1974, 1976), see Beck (1990). In short, the California Supreme Court determined that clinicians have a duty to take reasonable care to protect the foreseeable victims of dangerous patients. The onus is on the clinician to decide what is the most appropriate method of protection (e.g., by hospitalizing the patient, giving warnings by telephone and in writing to the foreseeable victim, informing the police, or refusing to release or discharge the patient). Jurisdictions differ in their interpretations of the breadth of this doctrine. Readers are advised to check on the precedents in their own states.

3. Circumstances in Which Malpractice Is Most Likely to Occur

a. Hospitalization

Malpractice is most likely to occur during the admission of a patient to a hospital if the practitioner negligently fails to admit a patient who requires hospital care, or if a patient is wrongfully or fraudulently committed to a hospital against his or her will. During treatment, negligence is most likely to occur if the hospital or physician fails to prevent a suicidal or assaultive patient from harming him- or herself or others, erroneously releases a patient dangerous to self or others, fails to protect an endangered third party (e.g., by warning that party that he or she is in danger of being harmed by a released or absconded patient), or subjects a patient to assault and battery (e.g., by overly vigorous restraint). The hospital may breach confidentiality or defame patients or others if it negligently discloses records.

b. Medication

Malpractice is most likely to occur during medication when the practitioner fails to obtain informed consent, fails to detect contraindications to the use of the drug (including previous adverse reactions), prescribes drugs that interact dangerously, fails to monitor the patient for side effects (e.g., tardive dyskinesia), or prescribes a drug that the patient subsequently uses to commit suicide.

c. Psychotherapy

During outpatient treatment, malpractice suits are most likely to arise when a clinician abandons an uncooperative patient without helping the patient find alternative care, fails to communicate adequately with a covering physician when away on vacation, recklessly inflicts emotional distress, breaches confidentiality, defames the patient, or sexually exploits the patient.

d. Teaching and research

Subjects may sue researchers or clinical teachers on the grounds of invasion of privacy, failure to obtain informed consent, or defamation. (For a fuller exposition of malpractice, see Nurcombe 1991; Holder 1991.)

E. JUVENILE DELINQUENCY

1. Definitions

"Juvenile delinquency" refers to juvenile offenses that would be subject to criminal sanctions if committed by adults. "Status offense" refers to unruly behavior subject to legal sanction in minors but not adults (e.g., curfew violation, disobedience, truancy, running away from home, or exposure to moral danger).

2. Legal Doctrines

Before the turn of the twentieth century, juvenile offenders were handled in a punitive manner. At that time, the legal system changed, and rehabilitation became the primary aim. During the 1960s, however, the rehabilitative model was toppled by the criticism of civil libertarians who likened juvenile justice to a "kangaroo court" (*In re Gault* 1967). At the same time, outraged by the surge of juvenile crime, many citizens claimed that benevolence had failed. As a consequence, the rehabilitative system was supplanted by a more legalistic system that aims at diversion, deinstitutionalization, and retribution (but which nevertheless retains vestiges of its more liberal forerunner).

The landmark cases that acted as a watershed in this change were *Kent v. United States* (1966), *In re Gault* (1967), *In re Winship* (1970), *McKeiver v. Pennsylvania* (1971), *Breed v. Jones* (1975), and *Fare v. Michael C.* (1979). In *Kent*, the Supreme Court held that, before he or she can be transferred to an adult court, a juvenile offender must be accorded due process; specifically, the juvenile must have counsel, a formal hearing, access to records, and a statement of the reason for the transfer. *Breed* established the requirement of a special hearing before transfer of a juvenile to adult court. In *Gault*, the Supreme Court held that the Bill of Rights and the Fourteenth Amendment applied to juvenile offenders, who therefore must be afforded counsel, advanced notice of the hearing, the right to cross-examine witnesses, protection from hearsay, and privilege against police interrogation without the support of a parent or guardian. *Winship* set the highest standard of proof for juveniles accused of offenses that might lead to loss of liberty ("beyond a reasonable doubt"). However, in *McKeiver,* the Supreme Court held that a jury was not constitutionally mandated for juveniles, and in *Fare* the Supreme Court determined that a juvenile might validly waive his *Miranda* rights (*Miranda v. State of Arizona* 1966).

In 1974, the federal government enacted the Juvenile Justice and Delinquency Prevention Act. This act aimed to foster prevention, obviate the placement of juveniles in adult jails, promote the diversion and treatment of juveniles, and decriminalize status offenses.

3. Legal Circumstances Requiring Mental Health Evaluation

Mental health clinicians are most likely to be asked to evaluate a juvenile offender before a dispositional hearing, before a transfer hearing, before adjudication, or before diversion. They will probably be asked to advise the court with regard to whether the offender has a disorder amenable to treatment, whether the offender is dangerous to self or others, whether there are mitigating circumstances, whether there are compelling reasons not to transfer a juvenile to adult court, and the most appropriate disposition and treatment for the offender. Less commonly, clinicians will be called on to evaluate a juvenile's competence to waive *Miranda* or due process rights, a juvenile's competence to stand trial, or his or her mental state at the time of an offense.

In conducting their evaluations, mental health professionals should be sensitive to sociocultural issues. Social differences between the clinician and the family or child can impede or distort the assessment process, particularly when mutual stereotyping intrudes. The clinician should become familiar with the dialect and terminology used by the ethnic group or subculture to which the interviewee belongs. Communication problems of this sort are particularly likely to arise during the evaluation of cases related to child maltreatment or neglect, juvenile delinquency, and mental health law. What, for example, is the Cambodian norm with regard to the punishment of children? Which are the dominant street gangs in the city? What terms do juvenile drug dealers and users employ? Are you able to follow an extreme black or Hispanic dialect? Before becoming involved in such cases, middle-class clinicians should familiarize themselves with the dialect, terminology, and sociocultural characteristics of the people involved.

a. Diagnosis

A forensic evaluation of use to the court must go beyond a mere categorical diagnosis. It should include an evaluation of the inherent and early psychosocial factors that predisposed the individual to delinquency, the stresses (if any) that precipitated the delinquency, the pattern of the offense or offenses, the environmental factors that reinforced or failed to prevent delinquency, the conscious and unconscious motivation of the delinquent act, and the offender's intelligence, capacity to learn, and prognosis with or without treatment.

b. Amenability

Is the juvenile willing or able to cooperate in rehabilitation or treatment? What is the likelihood of improvement?

c. Disposition

Possible dispositions include dismissal; probation; outpatient treatment; day treatment; placement in a residential treatment center, psychiatric hospital, correctional institution, or wilderness camp; and placement in a group or foster home. The disposition may involve specific mental health treatment, with or without provision for special medical, educational, or vocational needs.

d. Dangerousness

How dangerous is the youth likely to be to others (e.g., by virtue of assaultiveness, homicidal behavior, recklessness, or disturbed sexuality), to property (e.g., as a result of arson, vandalism, or recklessness), or to himself or herself (as a result of suicidality, self-injury, lack of self-care, physical or sexual provocativeness, or recklessness)?

e. Waiver to adult court

In determining whether a minor should be transferred to stand trial as an adult, judges take into account the offender's age, prior record, medical and psychiatric history, current medical and psychiatric status, and amenability to treatment, together with the seriousness of the offense, mitigating circumstances, the availability of treatment programs, and the safety of the public. Mental health clinicians can advise the court on several of these matters, particularly past history, current status, amenability to treatment, dangerousness, mitigating circumstances, and the suitability or availability of treatment programs.

f. Competence

See Curran et al. (1986), Grisso (1986), and Melton et al. (1983, 1987) for a fuller discussion of the evaluation of different kinds of competence in adults and minors. With regard to the waiving of rights by minors, the clinician must evaluate whether the juvenile did so voluntarily (i.e., uncoerced), knowingly (i.e., aware of the consequences), and intelligently (i.e., by weighing the pros and cons of the waiver).

g. Mental state at the time of the offense

This matter is unlikely to be at issue except when a juvenile is being tried for a serious crime in adult court, or when waiver to adult court is under consideration. For a fuller exposition of this complex (and controversial) matter, see articles and texts on forensic psychiatry (e.g., Dix 1984; Curran et al. 1986; Melton et al. 1987). Currently, in the United States, there are several legal standards for exculpation on grounds of legal insanity:

i. **The McNaughtan standard.** " . . . As a result of mental disease or defect, he was suffering from a defect in reason which caused him not to know either the nature and quality of the act or that the act was wrong."

ii. **Irresistible impulse.** " . . . As a result of mental disease or defect, he did not possess a will sufficient to restrain the impulse that may have arisen from his diseased mind."

iii. **The Model Penal Code, American Law Institute.** " . . . If, as a result of mental disease or defect, the defendant lacks substantial capacity either to appreciate the wrongfulness of his conduct or to conform his conduct to the requirements of the law."

iv. **Capacity to form specific intent.** Several states have replaced the insanity defense with a determination of whether the defendant had the capacity to form *mens rea,* that is, a specific intent to commit the crime.

v. **Guilty but mentally ill.** This standard does not exculpate the defendant.

h. **Mitigating factors**

Mitigation is most likely to be relevant to sentencing. The defense of diminished responsibility (e.g., due to intoxication, epileptic automatism, or dissociation) is introduced, rarely, with the aim of inducing the judge to reduce the sentence.

4. Research

For summaries of research into the epidemiology, sociology, typology, biology, family background, treatment, and prevention of juvenile offenders, see Farrington (1988), Garrett (1985), Gold (1987), Gottschalk et al. (1987), Lorion et al. (1987), Quay (1987a, 1987b, 1987c), Snyder and Patterson (1987), and Trasler (1987).

F. MENTAL HEALTH LAW

1. Legal Doctrines

The State derives its authority to confine mentally ill patients against their will from two doctrines: *police power* and *parens patriae*. Police power refers to the obligation of the State to protect its citizens from the dangerous behavior of others. Parens patriae refers to the State's responsibility to protect children and the mentally impaired. Due process refers to the obligation of the State to act fairly when it proposes to infringe on civil liberties. Due process checks and balances the State's police and paternalistic powers.

As with the juvenile justice system, mental health law has passed from an era of benevolence, during which the need for treatment was supported, to an era of legalism in which individual rights were emphasized. At the same time, the prevailing model of psychiatric hospitalization has been transformed from long-term custody or rehabilitation to short-term stabilization. The stabilization model aims to discharge patients early to less-restrictive treatment alternatives. In most states, in consequence of renewed emphasis on civil liberties, standards for civil commitment have changed from a medical model (i.e., "need for treatment") to a criminal model (i.e., "dangerousness").

Emergency commitment usually requires evidence that the patient is at imminent risk of serious harm or of harming others and that less restrictive treatment alternatives have failed or would be inadequate. Civil commitment typically requires a petition by two physicians that the patient is at serious risk of substantial harm and incompetent to make health care decisions. Readers should ascertain the criteria in their own states. The most important case in the field of child mental health is *Parham v. J.R.* (1979). This class action suit was brought on behalf of minors voluntarily admitted to mental hospitals on the application of their parents or guardians. It sought to replace Georgia's voluntary admission procedures for minors with a judicial adversary hearing. The Supreme Court disagreed, holding that the admitting physician, as "a neutral fact finder," was sufficient protection against improper admission. Thus adversary hearings were not required.

Other landmark cases were *Pennshurst State School and Hospital v. Haldeman* (1981) and *Youngberg v. Romeo* (1982). In these class action suits, the central issue was whether committed patients have a constitutional right to treatment. The Supreme Court rejected this argument, holding that the civilly committed residents of a state institution for the mentally retarded had a due process right to no more than safe conditions, freedom from unreasonable restraint, and minimum training to prevent deterioration or self-harm.

The extent to which the controversial right to refuse treatment applies to minors is unclear because the matter has never been adjudicated. Weithorn and Campbell (1982) discussed the competence of minors to decide for themselves whether they want treatment.

G. SUMMARY

Mental health clinicians are most likely to be asked to advise the courts in cases involving child custody disputes, allegations of child maltreatment, the termination of parental rights, civil liability, malpractice, juvenile delinquency, and mental health law. To be of help to the courts, it is essential that the forensic expert evaluate cases, provide reports, and testify in a manner relevant to the legal issues at stake. An appreciation of the legal doctrines and precedents that apply to these situations is, therefore, essential to clinicians who work in this area. It is also essential that expert witnesses be up to date with the most important research into the issues in question.

H. TABLE OF CASES AND LAWS

Alsager v District Court, 406 F Supp 10 (50 Iowa 1975)

In re Bachelor, 508 P 2d 862 (Kan 1973)

Battala v State of New York, 10 NY 2d 237 (1961)

Bezio v Patenande, 381 Mass 563, 410 NE 2d 1207 (1980)

Bloss v Bloss, 711 P 2d 663 (Ariz App 1985)

Breed v Jones, 421 US 519, 529 (1975)

Canterbury v Spence, 464 F 2d 772 (DC Cir 1973)

Christian v Randall, 33 Colo App 129, 516 P 2d 132 (1973)

Cobb v Grant, 8 Cal 3d 229, 502 P 2d 1, 104 Cal Rptr 505 (1971)

Ex parte Devine, 398 So 2d 686 (Ala 1981)

DiStefano v DiStefano, Go AD 2d 976, 401 NYS 2d 636 (1978)

Fare v Michael C, 442 US 707, 725 (1979)

Federal Adoption Assistance and Child Welfare Act, 42 USC Sect 601, 620, 670 (1980)

In re Gault, 387 US 1 (1967)

Harrison v Harrison, 359 So 2d 266 (La App 1978)

Johnson v Lundell, 361 NW 2d 125 (Minn App 1958)

Juvenile Justice and Delinquency Prevention Act of 1974, Pub L No 93-415, codified at 42 USC Sec 5601 et seq

In re K.B., 302 NW 2d 410 (SD 1981)

Kent v United States, 383 US 541, 544 (1966)

Landeros v Flood, 11 Cal 3d 399, 551 P 2d 389, 131 Cal Rptr 69 (1976)

Looper v McManus, 581 P 2d 487 (Okla 1978)

McIntyre v McIntyre, 452 So 2d 14 (Fla 1984)

McKeiver v Pennsylvania, 403 US 528 (1971)

Michigan Child Custody Act, Mich Comp Laws Ann 722 (1970)

Miranda v State of Arizona, 384 US 436, 86 S Ct 1062 (1966)

Palmore v Sidoti, 466 US 429 (1984)

Parham v J.R. 442 US 584 (1979)

Pennshurst State School and Hospital v Haldeman, 451 US 1 (1981)

Prince v Massachusetts, 321 US 158 (1944)

Pusey v Pusey, 728 P 2d 117 (1986)

Schloendorff v Society of New York Hospital, 211 NY 125, 105 NE 92 (1914)

State ex rel Watts v Watts, 77 Misc 2d 178, 350 NY 2d 285 (Sup Ct 1973)
State v Jones, 95 NC 588 (1856)
Tarasoff v Regents of the University of California, 529 P 2d 553, 118 Cal Rptr 129 (1974), 17 Cal 3d 425, 551 P 2d 334, 131 Cal Rptr 14 (1976)
Tobin v Grossman, 24 NY 2d 609 (1969)
Uniform Child Custody Jurisdiction Act, 9 ULA 103 (1968)
Uniform Marriage and Divorce Act, 9A ULA 91 (1970)
In re Winship, 397 US 358 (1970)
Witmayer v Witmayer, 467 A 2d 371 (Pa Super 1983)
Wrecsis b. Boughton 426 A2d 1155 (Pa Super 1981)
Youngberg v Romeo, 457 US 307 (1982)

I. REFERENCES

Beck JC: Clinical aspects of the duty to warn or protect, in Review of Clinical Psychiatry and the Law, Vol I. Edited by Simon RJ. Washington, DC, American Psychiatric Press, 1990, pp 191–204

Billingham RE, Saver AK, Pillion LA: Family structure in childhood and sexual attitudes and behaviors during late adolescence. Paper presented at the annual meeting of the National Council on Family Relations, New Orleans, LA, November 1989

Block J, Block JH, Gjerda PF: Parental function and the home environment in families of divorce. J Am Acad Child Psychiatry 27:207–213, 1988

Buchanan CM, Maccoby EE, Dornbusch SM: Caught between parents: adolescents' experience in divorced homes. Child Dev 62:1008–1029, 1991

Cicchetti D, Carlson V: Child Maltreatment: Theory and Research on the Causes and Consequences of Child Abuse and Neglect. New York, Cambridge, 1989

Curran WJ, McGarry AL, Shah SA: Forensic Psychiatry and Psychology: Perspectives and Standards for Interdisciplinary Practice. Philadelphia, PA, F. A. Davis, 1986

Dix GE: Criminal responsibility and mental impairment in American criminal law: response to the Hinckley acquittal in historical perspective, in Law and Mental Health: International Perspectives, Vol I. Edited by Weisstub DN. New York, Pergamon, 1984, pp 1–44

Farrington DP: Advancing knowledge about delinquency and crime: the need for a coordinated program of longitudinal research. Behavioral Sciences and the Law 6:307–331, 1988

Finkelhor D: Child Sexual Abuse: New Theory and Research. New York, Free Press, 1984

Finkelhor D, Browne A: The traumatic impact of child sexual abuse. Am J Orthopsychiatry 55:530–541, 1985

Furstenberg FF, Morgan SP, Allison P: Paternal participation and children's well-being after marital dissolution. Am Sociol Rev 52:695–701, 1987

Garrett CJ: Effects of residential treatment on adjudicated delinquents: a meta-analysis. Journal of Research in Crime and Delinquency 22:287–308, 1985

Glenn ND, Kramer KB: The psychological well-being of adult children of divorce. J Marriage Fam 47:905–912, 1987

Gold M: Social ecology, in Handbook of Juvenile Delinquency. Edited by Quay HC. New York, Wiley, 1987, pp 62–105

Gottschalk R, Davidson WS, Gensheimer LK, et al: Community-based interventions, in Handbook of Juvenile Delinquency. Edited by Quay HC. New York, Wiley, 1987, pp 266–289

Grisso T: Evaluating Competencies: Forensic Assessments and Instruments. New York, Plenum, 1986

Guidibaldi J: Differences in children's divorce adjustment across grade level and gender, in Children of Divorce. Edited by Wolchik S, Karoly P. Lexington, MA, Lexington Books, 1988, pp 185–231

Haugaard JJ, Reppucci ND: The Sexual Abuse of Children: A Comprehensive Guide to Current Knowledge and Intervention Strategies. San Francisco, CA, Jossey-Bass, 1988

Hetherington EM: Stress and coping in children and families, in Children in Families Under Stress (New Directions for Child Development, No 24). Edited by Doyle A, Gold D, Moskowitz DS. San Francisco, CA, Jossey-Bass, 1984, pp 7–33

Hetherington EM: Coping with family transitions. Child Dev 60:1–14, 1989

Hetherington EM, Clingempeel WG: Coping with marital transitions. Monographs of the Society for Research in Child Development 2–3. 57:1–242, 1992

Hetherington EM, Cox M, Cox R: Divorced fathers. Fam Coord 25:417–428, 1976

Hetherington EM, Cox M, Cox R: The aftermath of divorce, in Mother-Child, Father-Child Relationships. Edited by Stevens JH Jr, Mathews M. Washington, DC, National Association for the Education of Young Children, 1978

Hetherington EM, Cox M, Cox R: Play and social interaction in children following divorce. Journal of Social Issues 35:26–49, 1979

Hetherington EM, Stanley-Hagen M, Anderson ER: Marital transitions. Am Psychol 44:303–312, 1989

Holder AR: Issues in professional liability, in Child and Adolescent Psychiatry. Edited by Lewis M. Baltimore, MD, Williams & Wilkins, 1991, pp 1139–1144

Hutchens DJ, Kirkpatrick MJ: Lesbian mothers/gay fathers, in Emerging Issues in Child Psychology and the Law. Edited by Schetky DH, Benedek EP. New York, Brunner/Mazel, 1985, pp 115–126

Johnston JR, Campbell LEG: Impasses of Divorce. New York, Free Press, 1988

Kelly J, Wallerstein J: The effects of parental divorce: experiences of the child in early latency. Am J Orthopsychiatry 46:20–32, 1976

Lorion RP, Tolan PH, Wahler RG: Prevention, in Handbook of Juvenile Delinquency. Edited by Quay HC. New York, Wiley, 1987, pp 383–416

McFarlane AC: Posttraumatic phenomena in a longitudinal study of children following a natural disaster. J Am Acad Child Psychiatry 26:764–769, 1987

Melton GB, Koocher GP, Saks MJ: Children's Competence to Consent. New York, Plenum, 1983

Melton GB, Petrila J, Poythress NG, et al: Psychological Evaluations for the Courts: A Handbook for Mental Health Professionals and Lawyers. New York, Guilford, 1987

Nurcombe B: Malpractice, in Child and Adolescent Psychiatry. Edited by Lewis M. Baltimore, MD, Williams & Wilkins, 1991, pp 1127–1138

Nurcombe B, Ünützer J: The ritual abuse of children: diagnosis and forensic evaluation. J Am Acad Child Adolescent Psychiatry 30:272–276, 1991

Pynoos RS, Eth S (eds): Posttraumatic Stress Disorder in Children. Washington, DC, American Psychiatric Press, 1984

Quay HC: Institutional treatment, in Handbook of Juvenile Delinquency. Edited by Quay HC. New York, Wiley, 1987a, pp 244–265

Quay HC: Intelligence, in Handbook of Juvenile Delinquency. Edited by Quay HC. New York, Wiley, 1987b, pp 106–117

Quay HC: Patterns of delinquent behavior, in Handbook of Juvenile Delinquency. Edited by Quay HC. New York, Wiley, 1987c, pp 118–138

Senior N, Gladstone T, Nurcombe B: Child snatching: a case report. J Am Acad Child Psychiatry 21:579–583, 1983

Sgroi SM: Handbook of Clinical Intervention in Child Sexual Abuse. Lexington, MA, Lexington Books, D. C. Heath, 1982

Snyder J, Patterson GR: Family interaction and delinquent behavior, in Handbook of Juvenile Delinquency. Edited by Quay HC. New York, Wiley, 1987, pp 216–243

Terr LC: Childhood traumas: an outline and overview. Am J Psychiatry 148:10–20, 1991

Trasler G: Biogenetic factors, in Handbook of Juvenile Delinquency. Edited by Quay HC. New York, Wiley, 1987, pp 184–215

Walker LEA (ed): Handbook on Sexual Abuse of Children: Assessment and Treatment Issues. New York, Springer, 1988

Wallerstein J: Children of divorce: the psychological tasks of the child. Am J Orthopsychiatry 53:240–243, 1983

Wallerstein J, Kelly J: The effects of parental divorce: experiences of the pre-school child. J Am Acad Child Psychiatry 14:600–616, 1975

Wallerstein J, Kelly J: The effects of parental divorce: experiences of the child in later latency. Am J Orthopsychiatry 46:256–269, 1976

Wallerstein J, Kelly J: Effects of divorce on the visiting father-child relationship. Am J Psychiatry 137:1534–1539, 1980a

Wallerstein J, Kelly J: Surviving the Breakup: How Children and Parents Cope With Divorce. New York, Basic Books, 1980b

Wolchik S, Karoly P (eds): Children of Divorce: Perspectives on Adjustment. Lexington, MA, DC Heath, 1985

CHAPTER ELEVEN

The Forensic Evaluation

Barry Nurcombe, M.D.

T his chapter describes the principles and practice of forensic evaluation, from the initial contact with the attorney to the preparation of the forensic report. For the purposes of illustration, a civil liability case is described. The reader should apply the principles exemplified in this kind of case to the other situations discussed in Chapter 10.

A. THE EXPERT WITNESS

In law, a witness is somebody who has personally experienced an event and who subsequently testifies to what he or she has perceived. Thus, a clinician who has treated a client on certain dates may be called on to testify thereto, as a *fact witness*. In law, a fact refers to something that has actually occurred. Questions of fact are for the jury to decide; questions of law are for the judge to decide.

As described in Chapter 9 ("Types of Witnesses"), an *expert witness* is called on when the court needs technical information beyond the grasp of a layman. Before the expert is allowed to give testimony, the judge must qualify him or her as having an acceptable level of training and experience in the particular field. Whereas fact witnesses are not allowed to testify to hearsay or opinion, expert witnesses are permitted to make inferences, give opinions, testify to hearsay, and introduce "learned treatises" (e.g., scientific articles) into evidence. For example, in view of the fact that history taking is an accepted part of the diagnostic process, a hearsay history taken from a parent about a child may form part of a clinician's evidence concerning that child. The expert witness is also permitted to respond to hypothetical questions, in other words, to draw a professional conclusion assuming that certain facts are true. Expert opinion must be based on "reasonable probability" and be derived from procedures that are "well recognized" and "sufficiently established" to have gained "general acceptance" in the expert's field (*Frye v. United States* 1923). Thus, the mental health clinician has the responsibility of choosing diagnostic procedures that have adequate reliability and validity. Expert witnesses are entitled to higher fees than fact witnesses.

The role of the expert witness can be described according to the following set of maxims:

- *Be an informant, not an advocate.* It is impossible for the expert not to be affected in the adversary atmosphere of litigation. Before the trial, the lawyer who retains the expert may be eager to obtain a favorable opinion. Experts may find themselves inclined to side with children who have been harmed or with parents who are paying for an evaluation. During the trial, a vigorous cross-examination may tempt the expert to respond with partisan heat. Such pressures notwithstanding, the forensic expert should resist espousing causes, and strive to remain professionally balanced and unbiased. Attorneys, judges, and juries are most likely to be persuaded by witnesses who are unimpassioned, reasonable, and impartial. The wise expert will seek effective methods of advocating his or her opinion; however, in the long run, the purposes of the law are best served when the expert aims to provide reliable information for the court to cogitate. Lawyers advocate; experts inform.
- *Evaluate, don't treat.* It is inevitable that therapists will identify with their patients and, thus, be biased in their favor. Furthermore, testifying in court concerning a patient raises questions of confidentiality and double agentry, even when the patient has waived privilege (i.e., relinquished the right to keep confidential matters private). Therefore, avoid being an expert witness concerning your patients, unless this is unavoidable, and don't propose to treat those you have evaluated. If you do so, you run the

risk of being impugned as having a mercenary interest in the court's decision.

- *Thoroughness and clarity supersede vigor of advocacy.* Judges and juries are more likely to be persuaded by experts who are thorough. Pursue data relevant to a particular issue from several sources that cross-check with each other. Pay close attention to previous mental health, medical, educational, and police documentation. Follow a stepwise interpretation of the reliability and significance of data that converge on the issue at stake in the case. For example, in a child custody dispute, organize your report and your testimony in accordance with those elements of "the best interests of the child" that apply in the jurisdiction in which you work.

- *Don't doctor the information.* It is not legitimate for experts to oversimplify issues, delete facts or inferences that mitigate the force of their opinions, or claim greater certainty for their opinions than is justified. In a complicated field such as mental health, no case is "perfect." Flaws, inconsistencies, and evidential gaps are inevitable; it is preferable to identify and discuss them in your report so that the attorney involved can prepare an effective strategy.

- *Don't claim more certainty than the data allow.* The vigorous advocacy of attorneys and the heat of the adversary situation may tempt you to assert more confidence in your opinions than is warranted by the quality of the information you have gathered. You render the case, the law, and your profession a disservice if you do so. Be frank about the uncertainties in your data or opinions, and claim reasonable certainty only when it is merited.

- *Don't testify to the ultimate issue.* It is for the court to determine whether an individual is incompetent to parent a child, not guilty by reason of insanity, or responsible for negligently harming another person. The court decides whether a child has been maltreated or negligently injured by someone else, what is in the best interests of a minor, and whether a juvenile has committed an offense. The expert's task is to gather information relevant to the ultimate issue—in other words, data pertinent to the elements that constitute the legal issues—so that the court may reach a just conclusion. Ultimate issues pose questions of morality and social policy that are outside the province of professional expertise. Attorneys and judges will sometimes press you to exceed your authority by giving conclusive reports or testimony. Resist them.

B. THE EVALUATION

1. Initial Contact

The forensic expert is most likely to be contacted first by an attorney, or less commonly by a parent. It is necessary to ascertain the nature and circumstances of the litigation and to discuss with the attorney the legal issues at stake. Decide then, or after the first interview with the parent or parents, whether you have anything useful to contribute. Ascertain the date of the trial or hearing. Make sure there is adequate time to complete an evaluation, and determine whether you will be available at that time. If not, ask whether a continuance of the case would be possible.

If you decide to accept the case, discuss your fees with the attorney. In civil liability suits the attorney handles all expenses, working on a contingency fee. In other cases, the family, insurance company, child protective agency, or public defender is responsible for paying your fees. Unless your client is an insurance company, it is appropriate to ask for a retainer, with the balance to be paid on completion of the report, before the report is issued. Most forensic clinicians charge an hourly rate and include the time spent reading documents and preparing the report. It is not advisable to charge a fee that greatly exceeds your fee for nonforensic work. Discuss also your fee (and expenses, if any) for a court appearance. For example, you may charge per half-day or full day, depending on the attorney's estimate of how long your testimony will take. Given the nature of the case and the number of people involved, estimate the approximate cost of the evaluation and quote your fee for a court appearance. Indicate that you will contact the attorney or parent and ask for instructions on how to proceed if the expenses of the evaluation appear likely to exceed your estimate. Do not rely on assurances alone; if you are unfamiliar with the attorney, draw up a contract setting out your mutual obligations.

Ask the attorney to forward to you all relevant documents— informed consent forms for recovery of documents, mental health evaluations, medical evaluations, educational assessments, school records, other forensic reports, confessions, police and witness reports, affidavits, interrogations, depositions, and previous judicial decisions. If you are unfamiliar with the legal issue at stake, ask the attorney to send you copies of the relevant statutes or case precedents.

Send your curriculum vitae to the attorney, marking any entries that support your special expertise in the area for which you have been consulted. Also, prepare a summary vita that will guide the attorney in the questions he or she will ask you when you are being qualified in court (see Chapter 12, section D2, "Qualification"). Be frank about any problems. For example, are you fully qualified, board certified, or licensed to practice in your state? Have your license or hospital privileges ever been rescinded? Has a malpractice suit been decided against you, or is a malpractice suit outstanding? Have you been charged with or convicted of a criminal offense?

Sometimes, the clinician's first contact is by subpoena. A subpoena is most likely to be received when a patient has been evaluated or treated by the clinician. In that case, the clinician should ascertain whether his or her presence in court is requested as a fact witness or as an expert witness. A subpoena will also be issued after a forensic evaluation to confirm the date and place of the hearing.

A subpoena is a summons to appear in court issued by a court at the request of an attorney or agency, or commanded by a judge. A subpoena duces tecum requires the witness to bring specified documents (e.g., clinical records) into court. A subpoena compels the witness to appear in court, but not to testify unless he or she is required to do so by the court. Unless the patient has waived privilege, the witness should appeal to the judge before disclosing confidential information. Because of the potential legal dangers of this situation, a clinician who unexpectedly receives a subpoena should inform the patient and his or her attorney, ask for their advice, and consult his or her own attorney before the court appearance. The record should be reviewed for potentially deleterious information. Your attorney might petition the court for a protective order that seals the record against the disclosure of private but irrelevant material.

2. Initial Interview

Discuss the proposed evaluation with the child's parents. In effect, you are asking them to give informed consent to the diagnostic procedures they and their child will be exposed to. They are also giving consent for you to put into a report anything you deem of relevance to the case, to issue that report to the attorneys involved, and to have the report entered as evidence. Obtaining this consent is particularly important in custody litigation. It is seldom appropriate to interview only one parent in a custody dispute, unless expert opinion is required only on a limited matter (e.g., the mental health of one parent). When the comparative appropriateness of the parents as custodians is in question, both must be seen. If a parent or attorney seeks to have you interview one parent only, explain why such an interview would be ineffective and recommend either that the attorneys for both sides agree to have both parents (and any other persons who have an important relationship to the child) interviewed or that the court be petitioned to order a forensic evaluation of all the parties involved.

Describe to the parents the purpose of the evaluation, its relevance to the legal issue at stake, and the probable timing and duration of the different interviews. If psychological testing will be required, explain its nature and purpose. Make it very clear that the purpose of the evaluation is not to provide them or their child with treatment, but rather to provide information for the court.

3. Evaluation Questions

In a typical civil liability case involving a child who claims psychological injury, the following questions must be addressed:

a. Diagnosis

Does the child currently suffer from psychiatric disorder, psychosocial impairment, or educational disability?

b. Severity

How serious is the disorder, impairment, or disability?

c. Pattern

What is the pattern of the disorder, impairment, or disability? Is it consistent with psychological trauma? Is there evidence for posttraumatic stress disorder?

d. Causation

Was the alleged trauma psychologically traumatic to the child? Was the trauma directly related to the child's current disorder, impairment, or disability? If so, was it the sole factor, the major factor, a contributory factor, or a minor precipitating factor? Did the child experience other stresses that could have resulted in the current disorder?

e. Preexisting condition

Did the child suffer from a disorder, impairment, or disability before the trauma? If so, did the trauma aggravate the preexisting condition? Was the trauma the sole aggravating factor, the major aggravating factor, a contributory aggravating factor, or a minor aggravating factor?

f. Perpetuation

Is there evidence that the child's condition has been perpetuated by environmental factors such as parental anxiety, or artificially shaped by parental indoctrination?

g. Prognosis

What is the child's outlook, with or without treatment? Is the child's current condition likely to affect later psychological, social, educational, or occupational adjustment?

4. Evaluation Procedures

First, the parents should be interviewed to gather information about the child's development; family background; marital adjustment; parental mental health; the child's adjustment at home, school, and with peers before the trauma; the history of the trauma and its circumstances; the child's and the family's adjustment after the trauma; the child's past medical, mental health, and educational history; and the possibility that one or both parents have advertently or inadvertently perpetuated the child's problems. (Three 1 1/2-hour interviews.)

Next, the parents should independently complete Child Behavior Checklists (Achenbach and Edelbrock 1983), Minnesota Multiphasic Personality Inventories (Hathaway and McKinley 1983), and Family Inventories of Life Events (McCubbin et al. 1987) to assess the psychosocial adjustment of the child and parents and the exposure of the family to stressful events other than the trauma in question. (One to two 1 1/2-hour interviews.)

The child then should be interviewed to determine whether there is evidence of psychological disorder, social impairment, or educational disability. The child's version of the trauma should be ascertained. If the differentiation of the child's disorder is unclear, a structured diagnostic interview may be helpful when the subject is at least 10 years old. Of particular relevance is the child's description of intrusive memories, flashbacks, nightmares, or reenactments of the traumatic experience, together with avoidance, numbing, amnesia, and hyperarousal related to the experience. A series of playroom interviews may be required for younger children, with the use of toys and drawings to gather relevant information. (Three to four 1-hour interviews.)

Children should be referred for formal psychological testing with regard to intelligence, educational achievement, personality, and, if indicated, neuropsychological functioning. It is preferable to refer children to a psychologist who is prepared to evaluate them on the basis of no more than a description of the alleged trauma and specific questions (see section on "Evaluation Questions"). (Two 3-hour interviews.)

It can be useful to interview witnesses (e.g., teachers) who can describe the child's behavior before, immediately after, and subsequent to the alleged trauma. Teachers should be asked to complete the Child Behavior Checklist—Teacher Version (Achenbach and Edelbrock 1983). (One hour for each interview.)

An additional interview with the child or parent may be necessary to check discrepancies or fill gaps in the evaluation.

5. Elucidating the Questions

a. Diagnosis, severity, and pattern

Information concerning these issues is derived from the parental history, the interviews with the child, information from other informants (e.g., teachers), checklist data, and psychological testing. Does the child suffer from a disturbance, disorder, or disability? How sever is it? What is its pattern? Can it be assigned to a DSM-III-R category (American Psychiatric Association 1987)?

b. Causation

Was the alleged trauma actually traumatic to the child? Did the stress of the trauma precipitate the current disturbance, disorder, or disability? The impact of trauma is validated by informants who can describe the child's reaction at the time of the event, by police reports of the event, or by medical reports that describe the child's immediate reaction to the event. The onset of symptoms soon after an event supports its traumatic nature, although the diagnosis of a delayed stress reaction should be considered in some cases (e.g., when a subsequent stress reactivates a preexisting psychological trauma). The impact of the trauma is further evidenced in the quality of the symptomatology (e.g., repetitive dreams, intrusive memories, flashbacks, reenactments, traumatic play, amnesia for the incident, or avoidance of reminders of the trauma).

c. Aggravation

Did the alleged trauma aggravate a preexisting disorder? Information concerning any preexisting disorder can be obtained from parental history; from the children themselves, if they are 10 years old or older; from independent informants such as day-care providers or teachers; from previous mental health or pediatric reports; and from school records (before and after the alleged trauma).

d. Perpetuation

Evidence concerning inadvertent perpetuation can be derived from interviews with, and psychological testing of, the parents or guardians. It is not uncommon to find, for example, that a mother has sustained a posttraumatic stress reaction after seeing her child injured. The child's traumatic symptoms and the mother's stress reaction then interact in a vicious circle. Advertent perpetuation through parental indoctrination is suggested when the parental history does not match the child's, when the child's history is stilted and apparently rehearsed, and when psychological testing of the child does not match the parents' claims.

e. Prognosis and recommendations

The child's prognosis with or without treatment and the nature, probable duration, and costs of the recommended treatment are derived from published research and your personal experience. As previously discussed, avoid recommending yourself as the child's future therapist.

C. RECORDS

It is essential that the forensic clinician keep detailed, accurate records. All *telephone conversations* (e.g., with attorneys, parents, or mental health clinicians) should be dated, timed, and documented. All telephone messages should be dated, timed, and preserved in the record. Get into the habit of dating and timing all your notes. All too often, in the eyes of the law, if you didn't write it down, it didn't happen.

Blau (1984) provided a useful description of the documentary forms appropriate for forensic clinicians. An intake form should record the following: 1) the date and time of the initial contact with the attorney; 2) the attorney's name, address, and telephone number; 3) the names, addresses, and telephone numbers of the plaintiff, defendant, and the adversary attorney; 4) the facts of the case; 5) the issues at stake in the case; and 6) the anticipated date of the trial, the court, and the judge appointed to try the case. It is advisable for the attorney to sign a contract that obligates the clinician to undertake the evaluation and, if required, to prepare a forensic report in return for stipulated fees (see section B1, "The Initial Contact"). The clinician should use a standard informed consent form for gathering data and should keep copies of all requests for information sent to schools, hospitals, and other agencies or people.

The clinician will preserve all case notes taken during interviews with parents, children, and other informants and all audiotapes or videotapes taken during the evaluation. If the clinician is provided with a copy of another tape, the fact that it is a true copy should be documented by the person who copied it. Case reports, letters from agencies, and psychological test reports should be carefully filed. The psychologist should be careful to retain the raw data from which the report was derived.

The case record should be divided into tabbed sections, for example:

- A record of all interviews including time duration and charges
- The forensic evaluation report
- The initial contact sheet
- The contract

- Copies of the laws, statutes, regulations, or case precedents relevant to the case
- Scientific articles relevant to the case
- Legal records
- Medical, mental health, and school records
- Case notes
- Psychological test results
- Telephone messages
- Informed consent forms
- All letters to do with the case
- Audiotapes, videotapes, and so forth

D. THE FORENSIC EVALUATION REPORT

Before preparing a report, consult the attorney who has retained you. If your findings do not help the attorney's case, he or she may thank you, pay your fee, and ask you not to prepare a report. Clinicians must accept the narcissistic blow that their hard work will not always be of help. Because it is discoverable, an unfavorable report may be helpful to the other side's cause. Lawyers are quite within their right to ask you not to prepare a report; their task is to present the best possible argument for their clients. If an unfavorable report were prepared and a lawyer hid the fact, he or she would run the risk of being accused of withholding material evidence.

The reputation of forensic clinicians rests on their qualifications, the pertinence of the reports they prepare, and the quality of the testimony they give. A comprehensive, systematic, well-reasoned, relevant, and succinct evaluation report is essential to the attorney who is preparing a case and to the judge who tries it. Conversely, sloppy, disorganized, irrelevant, illiterate, jargon-ridden reports irritate judges and provide ammunition for adversary lawyers. Therefore, keep the following principles in mind:

- Proceed logically in your report from the issues at stake through the data elicited to your opinion and recommendations. In other words, describe the data before you analyze them and draw inferences.

- Eschew the passive voice; use the first person. A direct, personal style is more effective than circumlocutions.
- Avoid jargon, if possible. If you can't avoid it, define it. To describe a parent as having "borderline traits" conveys little to a lawyer. On the contrary, a moody and impulsive person with an unstable sense of identity and difficulty in sustaining close relationships is likely to be readily recognizable.
- Edit your manuscript closely. Winnow out all psychobabble (e.g., "meet the needs of the patient"), pomposities (e.g., "on the basis of . . . " and "in the process of . . . "), buzz words (e.g., "on the cusp" and "the cutting edge"), vogue usages ("the trauma impacted his personality"), and clichés.
- Avoid prolixity. Two sentences may be better than one.
- Prepare a double-spaced report. This spacing facilitates both editing and the recording of marginalia by attorneys and judges.

Organize the report headings, for example:

- *Identifying information.* The name, date of birth, and address of the primary subject or subjects of the report.
- *Circumstances of referral.* A brief description of the legal situation, nominating the attorney who referred the case.
- *Purpose of the evaluation.* List the legal and clinical issues addressed in the evaluation.
- *Informed consent.* Record that you have informed the parties involved that the evaluation is for forensic, not therapeutic, purposes; that anything disclosed or discovered may be included in a report for the attorneys involved and the court; and that the parties involved agreed to proceed with the evaluation.
- *Sources of data.* List the documents (with title, signature, and date), interviews (with subject, date, and duration of interview), tests (with subject, date, and tester), and other data from which your opinions and recommendations are derived.
- *Review of documents.* Summarize the documentary data relevant to the issues at stake.
- *Interviews.* Summarize the content of the interviews, using direct quotes whenever highly relevant matters are touched on. Summa-

rize your mental status observations as much as possible without using jargon. If you cannot avoid it, define it. For example:

> Mr. B described auditory hallucinations: every night, before he goes to sleep and when he is alone, he hears unfamiliar voices quarreling, berating him, or threatening to kill him. He is aware there is nobody in the room with him, and suggests that the voices may be transmitted by radio. He has no idea why this should be happening to him.

- *Psychological test results.* Summarize the test results with particular reference to the issues at stake. Include the full psychological test report in the appendix.
- *Discussion of findings.* Integrate the findings from different sources with reference to the issues. Point out and discuss the possible reasons for discrepancies between different data.
- *Summary and recommendations.* Using the issues as your guide, summarize your opinion. State first what you can aver with reasonable certainty (i.e., conclusions that would probably be reached by other clinicians with access to the data). State next those opinions that fall below the "reasonable certainty" standard. For example, you may say that particular behavior is consistent with (though not proof of) a child's having been sexually abused. Predict the range of future outcomes, acknowledging that a precise prognosis is not possible. Recommend the therapy required, discuss the likelihood of it being successful, and predict the range of time and cost likely to be required.
- *Appendixes.* Attach relevant transcripts of interviews, psychological test reports, and your curriculum vitae (indicating the training, experience, and publications relevant to your claim of expertise in this kind of case).

E. SUMMARY

The ultimate task of the forensic consultant is to provide reliable, expert information for the court to consider, information to which the court would not otherwise have access. Forensic consultants should be careful to rely on generally accepted diagnostic techniques of proven reliability. They should strive to avoid bias or even the appearance of partiality. Unless it is unavoidable, a therapist should not, for example, testify as an expert witness in a case involving someone he or she is treating. By the same token, forensic consultants should not proffer themselves as therapists for those they have evaluated.

No case is "perfect." There are always weaknesses in the information gathered. The forensic consultant should not withhold discrepant findings, delete data that are adverse to the case of those who have retained the consultant, or claim greater certainty than the data warrant. Thoroughness, clarity, and balance are more persuasive than partisanship. The expert witness should avoid testifying to ultimate issues; as matters of morality and social policy, they fall beyond the province of clinical expertise. The proper function of the expert is to advance the interests of justice by elucidating the legal questions at stake in the case.

The evaluation proper proceeds from the initial contact with the attorney, or from the receipt of a subpoena, through the review of documents, interviews, and psychological testing to the preparation of a forensic evaluation report. In addition, the expert witness should keep detailed case records and organize them in classified sections.

The forensic evaluation report should be edited to remove jargon, clichés, and vogue words. It should be written clearly and systematically, using headings. It should proceed from the circumstances of the referral, through the purpose of the evaluation, the sources of the data, a review of documents, and a summary of interviews and psychological test results, to a critical analysis of the findings. It should end with an opinion about the elements of the legal issue at stake and with recommendations for future treatment. The forensic evaluation report forms an important, sometimes crucial, part of the attorney's case, and it is likely to be entered into evidence for the judge or jury to consider. By the same token, an irrelevant, poorly organized report provides tempting ammunition for the other side to fire back in crossexamination.

F. SELECTED READINGS

In this chapter I chose a civil liability case as an example. For the evaluation of other legal issues, see R. S. Benedek and Benedek (1980) and Weiner et al. (1985) (child custody); Schetky and Slader (1980) (termination of parental rights); Derdyn (1980) (adoption); Lewis (1980), Petti (1980), and Sacks and Sacks (1980) (juvenile delinquency and status offenses); E. P. Benedek (1985) (waiver of juveniles to adult court); E. P. Benedek and Schetky (1985) and Schetky and Green (1988) (allegations of sexual abuse); and Burlingame and Amaya (1985) (mental health law).

G. TABLE OF CASES AND LAWS

Frye v United States, 293 F 1013 (DC Cir 1923)

H. REFERENCES

Achenbach TM, Edelbrock CS: Manual for the Child Behavior Checklist and Revised Child Behavioral Profile. Burlington, VT, Queen City Printers, 1983

American Psychiatric Association: Diagnostic and Statistical Manual of Mental Disorders, 3rd Edition, Revised. Washington, DC, American Psychiatric Association, 1987

Benedek EP: Waiver of juveniles to adult court, in Emerging Issues in Child Psychiatry and the Law. Edited by Schetky DH, Benedek EP. New York, Brunner/Mazel, 1985, pp 180–190

Benedek EP, Schetky DH: Allegations of sexual abuse in child custody and visitation disputes, in Emerging Issues in Child Psychiatry and the Law. Edited by Schetky DH, Benedek EP. New York, Brunner/Mazel, 1985, pp 145–158

Benedek RS, Benedek EP: Participating in child custody cases, in Child Psychiatry and the Law. Edited by Schetky DH, Benedek EP. New York, Brunner/Mazel, 1980, pp 59–70

Blau TH: The Psychologist as Expert Witness. New York, Wiley Interscience, 1984

Burlingame WV, Amaya M: Psychiatric commitment of children and adolescents: Issues, current practices, and clinical impact, in Emerging Issues in Child Psychiatry and the Law. Edited by Schetky DH, Benedek EP. New York, Brunner/Mazel, 1985, pp 229–249

Derdyn AP: Adoption, in Child Psychiatry and the Law. Edited by Schetky DH, Benedek EP. New York, Brunner/Mazel, 1980, pp 119–138

Hathaway SR, McKinley JC: The Minnesota Multiphasic Personality Inventory Manual. New York, Psychological Corporation, 1983

Lewis DO: Diagnostic evaluation of the delinquent child: Psychiatric, psychological, neurological, and educational components, in Child Psychiatry and the Law. Edited by Schetky DH, Benedek EP. New York, Brunner/Mazel, 1980, pp 139–155

McCubbin HI, Patterson JM, Bauman LH, et al: Adolescent-Family Inventory of Life Events and Changes (A-FILE). St. Paul, MN, Family Social Science, 1987

Petti TA: The juvenile murderer, in Child Psychiatry and the Law. Edited by Schetky DH, Benedek EP. New York, Brunner/Mazel, 1980, pp 194–206

Sacks HS, Sacks HL: Status offenders: emerging issues and new approaches, in Child Psychiatry and the Law. Edited by Schetky DH, Benedek EP. New York, Brunner/Mazel, 1980, pp 156–193

Schetky DH, Green AH: Child Sexual Abuse: A Handbook for Health Care Professionals. New York, Brunner/Mazel, 1988

Schetky DH, Slader DL: (1980). Termination of parental rights, in Child Psychiatry and the Law. Edited by Schetky DH, Benedek EP. New York, Brunner/Mazel, 1980, pp 107–118

Weiner BA, Simons VA, Cavanaugh JL Jr: The child custody dispute, in Emerging Issues in Child Psychiatry and the Law. Edited by Schetky DH, Benedek EP. New York, Brunner/Mazel, 1985, pp 59–75

CHAPTER TWELVE

Giving Testimony as an Expert Witness

Barry Nurcombe, M.D.

This chapter describes the way in which a forensic consultant prepares to give testimony. Furthermore, it describes depositions, trials, and the task of being an expert witness in court. To be effective, the consultant must understand the culture of the courtroom, the function of those who take part in the legal drama, and the different constraints under which they operate. Despite the twists and turns of adversary attorneys, the consultant should keep in mind the ultimate purpose of giving testimony: to provide the court with reliable information and opinions that are relevant to the legal issues at stake in the case and that are unavailable to nonexperts.

A. THE PRETRIAL CONFERENCE

It is sometimes impossible to schedule a pretrial conference, particularly when overworked state protective agency attorneys are involved. Nevertheless, the forensic consultant should always try to arrange one. Without such a meeting, the attorney will have difficulty preparing an effective strategy for getting the best from the witness, and the witness will have little guidance in understanding the probable sequence of questions, those aspects of the testimony that require particular emphasis, and the lines of attack likely to be adopted by the cross-examining attorney.

At the pretrial conference, the consultant and the attorney can review the legal theory involved in the case and the way in which the consultant's testimony will bear on it. The potential flaws, discrepancies, and limitations in the expert's evaluation can be frankly discussed so that the attorney can prepare a strategy to cope with them. To take the wind out of the cross-examiner's sails, the attorney may decide to bring out the inevitable weaknesses in the expert's argument during direct examination. For example, in a civil liability suit, the forensic clinician may have found that a child had signs of an emotional disorder before an alleged trauma. The plaintiff's attorney might decide to have the clinician discuss these signs at the outset, before proceeding to elaborate on evidence that the preexisting disorder worsened after the trauma.

The attorney will familiarize the witness with the sequence of questions to be put in direct examination. As a rule, these questions flow in the following order: the qualification of the witness, the diagnostic investigations carried out, the findings of the evaluation, and the expert's opinion. Thus, testimony converges on the ultimate legal issue but stops before preempting the final conclusion (see Chapter 9 and Chapter 11).

The wise attorney does not rehearse the expert witness—spontaneous responses are much more persuasive than scripted recitations. However, the expert can assist the attorney by preparing a summary of his or her formal education, professional qualifications, professional appointments, clinical and forensic experience, scientific research, and publications. This summary is more helpful to the attorney than an unedited curriculum vitae. It should be appended to the curriculum vitae in the forensic evaluation report (see Chapter 11).

The attorney will define for the consultant the local standard for "reasonable (medical, clinical, professional, or scientific) certainty." This explanation will help the consultant decide whether it is possible to testify to a particular opinion with sufficient certainty. If not, the expert witness may be able to do no more than testify to a consistency between the data and a particular inference. For example, the expert may be able to state: "Taking all these findings together, it is my opinion, with reasonable clinical certainty, that this child has suffered a severe psychological injury as a result of sexual abuse." A less trenchant opinion might be as follows: "It is my opinion that the findings are consistent with the inference that this child has been psychologically damaged as a result of sexual abuse; however, there are other plausible explanations." "Reasonable certainty" refers, in most jurisdictions, to a "more likely than not" level of confidence, or to an opinion that would be reached by most other expert practitioners. In practice, the term is somewhat elastic: it falls short of absolute confidence but debars speculation. The expert should ask the attorney where along this continuum the local standard falls. Is the standard at a "preponderance" (51%), a "clear and convincing" (75%), or "beyond a reasonable doubt" (90%) level of confidence?

The attorney should prepare the witness for the cross-examiner's probable line of questioning. The interests and idiosyncrasies of the judge assigned to the case can also be discussed. Is he or she hostile to mental health experts, irritated by jargon, or interested in the psychology of legal matters? Will the judge expect the expert to testify to the ultimate issue or be offended if he or she does so?

Finally, the clinician should check the time of appearance (e.g., 8:30 A.M. or 2:00 P.M.), the probable duration of the testimony, the location of the courtroom, and where to go to announce that he or she has arrived. In most cases, the clinician should schedule either a half-day or a full day, depending on the nature of the case.

A conference is also recommended before a deposition. The attorney should explain the purpose of the deposition, outline the probable sequence of questions, and advise the expert on whether certain information should be removed from the files. Materials to do with the attorney's "work product" (i.e., papers concerning the attorney's legal strategy) are not discoverable by the other side.

B. PREPARING TO BE DEPOSED OR TO GIVE TESTIMONY IN COURT

Shortly before you give testimony at a deposition or in court, prepare your document and your mind, as follows:

1. Organize your files into sections in chronological order (see Chapter 11, section C, "Records"). Judges and juries are distracted by the witness who riffles through loose pages to locate an elusive document or fact.

2. Prepare a flow chart of the case that sets out the salient dates and events and put it at the front of the file.

3. Put your evaluation report close to the front of the case record so that you may refer readily to the dates and duration of your diagnostic procedures and the documents you reviewed before preparing the report.

4. Review and file all documents concerning the legal issues at stake.

5. Review and file relevant research and clinical literature. If you have published on the matter involved, read your own material. The cross-examiner who has read your work will be particularly eager to find discrepancies between your publications and your opinion in the case in question.

6. Prepare yourself for a "learned treatise" attack (see section on "Cross-Examination") by reviewing the literature that depreciates the reliability or validity of clinical opinion in the area involved (i.e., Ziskin and Faust 1988). Prepare a counterargument if one can be sustained.

7. Prepare any charts or illustrations that will help to convey the meaning of your testimony.

8. Check that the case has not been settled out of court or continued (i.e., postponed). Sometimes, the attorney will have forgotten to tell you, or the message will have gone astray.

C. DEPOSING

The term "discovery" refers to procedures whereby one party obtains from the adversary party information required in preparation for a trial. Discovery procedures involve gaining access to documents, health reports, and health records; the posing of interrogatories (see Chapter 9, section E3, "Civil Court Proceedings," Chapter 9); and the deposition of witnesses.

A deposition is the taking and recording of sworn testimony from a witness (the deponent) either for the purpose of discovery or to obtain evidence from somebody who cannot appear in court (for example, if the case is to be tried in another state). A deposition is usually conducted in an attorney's chambers or in the clinician's office. It is attended by the witness, the opposing attorneys, and a court reporter (although sometimes the proceedings are recorded on audiotape or videotape for later transcription). Aside from its function in discovery, a deposition allows an attorney to size up a witness and "go fishing" for flaws in the other side's case. Although the formal procedures that characterize court testimony appear to be somewhat relaxed at a deposition, be careful. A jocular atmosphere can tempt the unwary into uncorseted statements that are resurrected as evidence at the trial. Treat a deposition as you would a court appearance.

The deponent is first sworn. He or she is then qualified and subjected to direct examination. Next, the adversary lawyer conducts a cross-examination that is followed by redirect examination and re-cross-examination. During the deposition, the attorneys may object to particular questions as they would in open court; their objections are ruled on at a later date. If an objection is subsequently sustained, the relevant section of the deposition transcript will be erased. Finally, the adversary attorney is provided with access to the deponent expert's files. Any elements of the retaining attorney's "work product" (i.e., legal memoranda, impressions, discussions of legal theory, and witnesses' statements prepared by the attorney in anticipation of litigation) should have been removed from the files before the deposition, because they are not subject to discovery. The deponent is under no obligation to help the adversary attorney to organize, sort through, or interpret the files.

After the deposition has been transcribed, the forensic consultant should read it very carefully, correcting any errors with signed marginal comments. Do not sign the transcript without reading it; the inadvertent omission of the word "not," for example, can have you expressing ideas that are the reverse of your actual opinion. Such blunders may come back to haunt you in the trial. Consider, for example:

Counsel: You now say that Mr. C is not below average intelligence. In this deposition (*holding the document up and pointing at it*), you say he is below average intelligence. Is he or is he not below average? Just what do you believe, Doctor?

Make sure you have a copy of the deposition in your files. Reread it carefully before going to court.

D. TESTIFYING

1. Preparing to Testify

A trial is a serious business. Dress accordingly, men in suits and sober shirts, women in suits and tailored blouses. Avoid gold chains, jangling jewelry, flashy ties, leisure suits, pant suits, sports jackets, blazers, two-tone shoes, and open-toed sandals. Any clothing or ornament that could distract the judge and jury from listening to what you say is out of place.

When you arrive at the court, announce yourself to the judge's secretary or to the bailiff, who will tell you where to wait. Don't barge into the courtroom until you are invited to enter; if you overhear other witnesses, you run the risk of being "contaminated" by them. The judge could then declare a mistrial and hold you in contempt.

The courtroom is generally arranged with the judge's bench raised above the rest of the room. Usually the jury box is square on and to the right of the judge. At separate tables sit the prosecutor or the plaintiff and his or her attorney, the defendant and his or her attorney, the court reporter, the clerk of the court, bailiffs. Seats are provided for spectators. The witness box is usually to the right of the judge. However, in juvenile court, the witness often faces the judge between the opposing attorneys' tables.

The bailiff will tell you when to enter the courtroom. On doing so, go directly to the witness box, acknowledge the judge with a nod, face the clerk, and raise your hand. The clerk will then swear you in. Answer "I do" to the time-honored question, take your seat, and put your file on the surface in front of you.

2. Qualification

Next, the attorney conducting the direct examination will qualify you. If your credentials are exceptional, opposing counsel may seek to stipulate to your qualification to prevent the judge or jury from being impressed by them. The direct examiner would be wise to insist that your credentials be heard. For example:

Counsel: Please state your name and address.

Witness: James William South, 10 Lygon Place, Nashville, Tennessee 37212.

Counsel: Where did you receive your basic medical qualifications?

Witness: I graduated Doctor of Medicine from . . . Medical School, in 1970.

Counsel: Where did you receive your internship and residency training?

Witness: I undertook my internship and residency in general psychiatry at . . . Hospital from 1975 to 1978 and completed 2 years of child and adolescent psychiatry training at the same hospital in 1979 and 1980.

Counsel: What other professional qualifications do you have?

Witness: I am board certified in general psychiatry and child and adolescent psychiatry. I am a member of the American Psychiatric Association and the American Academy of Child and Adolescent Psychiatry.

Counsel: What professional appointments have you had?

Witness: I have been in the private practice of child and adolescent psychiatry since 1981. I was appointed clinical assistant professor of child psychiatry at . . . in 1981. I became clinical associate professor of . . . . I am currently . . . .

Counsel: What medicolegal experience have you had?

Witness: Since 1984, I have evaluated about 10 legal cases per year and have given testimony in about half that number, in the states of [state name] and [state name]. Most of my evaluations and testimony have been in the areas of child sexual abuse, child custody disputes, and civil liability litigation.

Opposing counsel may challenge your qualifications on the grounds of inadequate training or professional experience, insufficient expertise in the legal area involved in the case, lack of medical training, or the lack of ability of any mental health professional to give a reliable opinion on the legal issue in question. Psychologists must learn to stand their ground against the "lack of medical training" ploy. Obviously, if a question involves detailed knowledge of pharmacotherapy, a psychologist should disclaim expertise; just as a psychiatrist should decline to testify about the details of psychological testing. On the other hand, the skills required to evaluate an allegation of sexual abuse depend on postgraduate training and experience, not on basic professional training. Attacks on the competence of mental health professionals in general usually follow the "learned treatise" approach. It is for the judge to decide whether the challenge to your qualifications will be sustained.

3. Direct Examination

According to the sequence already outlined for you in the pretrial conference, the direct examiner will ask questions such as the following:

1. Who referred the case to you?
2. What was the purpose of the referral?
3. What interviews did you carry out? On what dates? And for what duration?
4. Please state your findings.
5. What tests or special investigations did you (carry out, arrange)?
6. Please summarize the findings.
7. What, then, is your opinion with reasonable (medical and professional) certainty?

When stating your findings, summarize the main points derived from the document review, interviews, and tests; reserve direct quotes for observations that are particularly telling or illustrative of your main points. Use DSM-III-R diagnoses (American Psychiatric Association 1987) when it is important to indicate that the person in question has a significant emotional disorder, but be prepared to define the disorder in terms of the person's symptoms and signs. Do not speculate unless the attorney asks you to do so and the question is not objected to; in that case, emphasize that you are speculating.

4. Cross-Examination

Remember that you are not an advocate for one side or another, but rather an impartial informant who has the task of conveying a reliable opinion. Do not overstate your opinion or claim greater certainty than the data allow. When counsel pose their questions to you, look at them, pause to be sure you understand, and then turn and deliver your answer to the judge or the jury, depending on which is the finder of facts (see Chapter 9, section E1, "Criminal Proceedings"). The slight pause has two advantages: it prevents you from dropping into a lulling and deceptive rhythm set by the cross-examiner, and it allows the attorney who retained you to object, if indicated, before you blurt out a damaging response. Visual aids such as charts and diagrams can be helpful in explaining technical matters. Metaphors and similes can also be useful in conveying technical concepts to a jury.

The cross-examiner may want you to give "yes" and "no" answers. Do so if it is appropriate to do so. If, in your opinion, a monosyllabic answer would distort the facts, say so. You may appeal to the judge in this manner:

Witness: Your Honor, a yes or no answer to this question would oversimplify a complex matter. Could I be permitted to explain the matter in more detail?

Judge: No, Dr. Smith, just answer counsel's question.

or

Judge: Go ahead, Doctor, expand on your answer.

Inexperienced witnesses fear the Perry Mason lawyer who stands over them hissing questions, waggling a forefinger in their faces, and reducing them to white-lipped stammering. Actually, this kind of harassment is uncommon, and it often means that the attorney is desperate. The confident counsel impugns his or her opponent's case; the counsel who is unsure what to do attacks the witness or beats the table. The counsel who hectors witnesses is likely to be objected to, to be told by the judge to tone down his or her questions, or to incur the hostility of the jury. Fear, rather, the courteous inquisitor who leads you gently down a garden path before springing a set trap (e.g., by dredging up something from the deposition transcript or from your own scientific publications that is inconsistent with your courtroom testimony). However trying the inquisition, avoid gratuitous comments, eschew ill-advised essays at humor, and resist the temptation to score off the cross-examiner. If you don't know the answer to a question, say "I don't know." The unruffled, reasonable, transparently impartial witness is the most persuasive.

Avoid jargon. If you must use it, define it at once, perhaps using metaphor or simile to convey the technical meaning. For example:

Witness: Ms. D suffers from a bipolar affective disorder. By this I mean that she is subject to manic episodes lasting up to 3 months, associated with greatly elevated mood and excitement, speeded-up thinking, and reckless spending and personal behavior. At other times, she has suffered from episodes of severe depressive mood. In between these periods of excitement and depression she is in good control of her life. Since she was 20 years of age, she has had three episodes of mania and two episodes of depression.

Other ploys aimed at rattling the witness are to take material out of context or to use incomplete quotes from the report or deposition. That is why it is very important to review the report and deposition thoroughly before appearing in court. The cross-examiner may sometimes attempt to trivialize your diagnostic techniques, for example, by referring to an interview as a "chat" or by describing probabilistic reasoning as "guesswork." Do not let the cross-examiner get away with it.

Counsel: So, your diagnosis was based on a chat with the patient?

Witness: No. It was based on a systematic psychiatric interview, a mental status examination, a review of past documents, the results of special investigations, and my experience with other cases of a similar nature.

A well-prepared attorney may try to trip you up on a technical question (e.g., the elements of a DSM-III-R diagnosis).

Counsel: Well, what *are* the criteria for diagnosing posttraumatic disorder?

Witness: Patients with posttraumatic stress disorder have experienced a severe stress after which they develop unbidden memories of the event that they can't get out of their heads, repeated nightmares of the event, flashbacks to the event, and reenactments of the event. . . .

An attorney bankrupt of ideas may be reduced to depicting you as a "hired gun."

Counsel: Doctor, how much are you being paid for your opinion?

Witness: I am paid on an hourly basis for my evaluation and the preparation of my report. I am paid on a half-day basis for a court appearance. My fee for a court appearance depends on how long I am kept in court.

An interesting cross-examination technique was described by Ziskin and Faust (1988) in *Coping with Psychiatric and Psychological Testimony.* This three-volume text reviews in great detail all the literature that casts doubt on the scientific status of psychology and psychiatry, the validity of psychiatric classification, the reliability of clinical diagnosis and psychological testing, the capacity of clinicians to detect simulation or malingering, and the relevance of forensic expertise to professional education, board certification, and clinical experience. The attorney using this cross-examination technique—the "learned treatise" attack—begins by referring to a book or article, seeking to have you agree that it is authoritative. You should avoid doing so. A single article is seldom the last word on any scientific matter, and textbooks are usually several years out of date by the time they are published.

Counsel: Dr. Smith, are you familiar with an article by D. L. Rosenhan published in 1983, entitled "On Being Sane in Insane Places"?

Witness: Yes.

Counsel: Do you agree that the article is an authoritative one?

Witness: No.

Counsel: Why not?

Witness: Because the article is based on poorly performed research and its conclusions are unjustified.

It is important, therefore, to be up to date with the most important critical articles in the field in question and to be able to rebut the arguments of these articles if it is possible. Poythress (1980) summarized counterarguments useful to a witness who is being "Ziskinized." Once attorneys become embroiled in the to-and-fro of learned debate, they are likely to get out of their depth very quickly and to lose the attention of the jury.

Hypothetical questions may be put by either side. The purpose of a hypothetical question is to have the witness draw an inference or conclusion from a specified set of assumptions. The direct examiner may pose a hypothetical question to emphasize the data elicited by the clinician and to reinforce the clinician's opinion. When cross-examiners pose hypothetical questions, their purpose is to suggest alternative premises and, therefore, the possibility of an opinion other than that put forward by the witness. If the attorney introduces premises that you have not elicited or with which you disagree, it is legitimate to point that out; nevertheless, you must answer the question.

Witness: Well, it's difficult for me to picture such a situation because, in this case, I did not find W, X, or Y. However, if W, X, or Y had been present, one possible conclusion would be Z.

5. Reexamination

The redirect examination is likely to be brief. In it, counsel will probably attempt to repair any damage done during the cross-examination and to have the witness reemphasize the main points of the testimony. In the recross-examination, counsel is not permitted to introduce new matters; only material already discussed in the direct examination and cross-examination may be discussed. The counsel's purpose is to underline weaknesses in the witness's expertise or argument and to suggest alternative explanations for the data.

6. Termination

When the examinations are complete, you will be excused. Gather up your impedimenta, thank the judge, nod to the jury, and exit by the door of entry. Do not linger in the courtroom listening to further proceedings; as a busy professional, you need to get back to your patients. Judges and juries are not impressed by clinicians who appear to be creatures of the courts.

E. SUMMARY

This chapter offers to convey practical advice to the clinician who is anticipating giving testimony. Preparation is the key to being an effective expert witness. At a pretrial conference, the clinician and the attorney will discuss the clinician's findings and opinion, reviewing the legal theory related to the case and the relevance of the forensic evaluation to the legal issues at stake. The clinician and the attorney will discuss weaknesses and flaws in the evaluation, enabling the attorney to prepare a strategy to deflect a counterattack from adversary counsel. The attorney will outline the sequence of questions in the direct examination, with particular reference to the expert's qualifications.

Shortly before giving testimony in a deposition or in open court, the expert should organize the case file; prepare a time-based flow chart of the case; review the file, the legal issues, and relevant scientific articles; prepare for a "learned treatise" attack; prepare any charts or illustrations; and check the date of the hearing.

Depositions should be attended with the formality and professionalism associated with a court appearance. Their purpose is to enable the opposing side to discover the other side's case and to prepare a strategy to counter it. The consultant should read the deposition transcript carefully, correcting any errors before signing the document.

Be careful not to enter the courtroom after arriving at the court. Court officials will tell you where to wait. After entering the courtroom, stand to be sworn, sit in the witness box, and attend to the attorney questioning you, but direct your answers to the triers of fact—the jury or the judge. You will first be qualified, a process for which you and the direct examiner will have prepared. You will then be asked to describe the circumstances of the referral; the purpose of the evaluation; the documents, interviews, and other investigations that formed the source of your data; and your findings. You will finally be asked to state your opinion "with reasonable certainty."

The cross-examiner will seek to find flaws in your qualifications, techniques, findings, or opinion, or in the competence of mental health clinicians in general. In redirect examination, counsel will seek to repair any damage and to reemphasize your salient points. In re-cross-examination, the adversary counsel will attempt to reemphasize any flaws or deficiencies in your qualifications, techniques, findings, or profession.

Attorneys are bound to emphasize the strengths of their own case while attempting to expose the weaknesses of the other side's case. There is a playlike quality to the adversary process and a certain amount of simulated bristling between the antagonists. Actually, the clinician may be surprised to find that warring advocates are the best of friends after the trial. In one sense, a trial is a game, albeit a serious one. In the midst of the crossfire and afterwards, clinicians would do well to maintain their objectivity and sense of proportion. Calm good sense blunts the sharpest attack.

F. SELECTED READINGS

Most textbooks on forensic psychology or forensic psychiatry contain sections on giving testimony. *The Psychologist as Expert Witness*

(Blau 1984) contains excellent descriptions of how to file records, prepare for court, and give testimony. *Psychological Evaluations for the Courts* (Melton et al. 1987) contains useful discussions of the expertise of mental health professionals, the ethical dilemmas confronting experts, report writing, and the advisability of refusing to testify to the ultimate issue in the case. *Clinical Handbook of Psychiatry and the Law* (Gutheil and Appelbaum 1991) contains excellent descriptions of the adversary system and the courtroom experience. For insight into how the other half thinks, *Coping with Psychiatric and Psychological Testimony* (Volumes I, II, and III) by Ziskin and Faust (1988) is essential reading. Do not overlook the instructive courtroom transcripts in Volume III of this work.

G. REFERENCES

American Psychiatric Association: Diagnostic and Statistical Manual of Mental Disorders, 3rd Edition, Revised. Washington, DC, American Psychiatric Association, 1987

Blau TH: The Psychologist as Expert Witness. New York, Wiley-Interscience, 1984

Gutheil TG, Appelbaum PS: Clinical Handbook of Psychiatry and the Law. New York, McGraw Hill, 1991

Melton GB, Petrila J, Poythress NG, et al: Psychological Evaluations for the Courts: A Handbook for Mental Health Professionals and Lawyers. New York, Guilford, 1987

Poythress NG: Coping on the witness stand: learned responses to "learned treatise." Professional Psychology 11:133–139, 1980

Ziskin J, Faust D: Coping with Psychiatric and Psychological Testimony, Vols I, II, and III. Marina del Rey, CA, Law and Psychology Press, 1988

Index

*Page numbers printed in **boldface** type refer to tables or figures.*